Molecular Pathology
(PCRs & IHC)

Molecular Pathology (PCRs & IHC)

Ramnik Sood MD (Pathology) Gold Medalist

Director
Specialty Diagnostic Labs, Goa
Consultant "A", Consultant Pathologist, Molecular Pathologist
Cytohistopathologist, UAE

Deepak G Tripathi BSc (Chemistry) MMS

Group President, Tulip Diagnostics Pvt. Ltd.
Former President
Association of Diagnostics Manufacturers of India (ADMI)

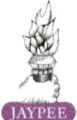

JAYPEE BROTHERS MEDICAL PUBLISHERS
The Health Sciences Publisher
New Delhi | London

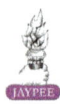

Jaypee Brothers Medical Publishers (P) Ltd

Headquarters
Jaypee Brothers Medical Publishers (P) Ltd
EMCA House, 23/23-B
Ansari Road, Daryaganj
New Delhi 110 002, India
Landline: +91-11-23272143, +91-11-23272703
+91-11-23282021, +91-11-23245672
Email: jaypee@jaypeebrothers.com

Overseas Office
J.P. Medical Ltd
83 Victoria Street, London
SW1H 0HW (UK)
Phone: +44 20 3170 8910
Fax: +44 (0)20 3008 6180
Email: info@jpmedpub.com

Corporate Office
Jaypee Brothers Medical Publishers (P) Ltd
4838/24, Ansari Road, Daryaganj
New Delhi 110 002, India
Phone: +91-11-43574357
Fax: +91-11-43574314
Email: jaypee@jaypeebrothers.com

EU GPSR Authorised Representative
LOGOS EUROPE, 9 rue Nicolas Poussin
17000, LA ROCHELLE, France
Phone: +33 (0) 6 67 93 73 78
Email: Contact@logos europe.eu

Website: www.jaypeebrothers.com
Website: www.jaypeedigital.com

© 2024, Jaypee Brothers Medical Publishers

The views and opinions expressed in this book are solely those of the original contributor(s)/author(s) and do not necessarily represent those of editor(s) and publisher of the book.

All rights reserved. No part of this publication may be reproduced, stored or transmitted in any form or by any means, electronic, mechanical, photocopying, recording or otherwise, without the prior permission in writing of the publishers.

All brand names and product names used in this book are trade names, service marks, trademarks or registered trademarks of their respective owners. The publisher is not associated with any product or vendor mentioned in this book.

Medical knowledge and practice change constantly. This book is designed to provide accurate, authoritative information about the subject matter in question. However, readers are advised to check the most current information available on procedures included and check information from the manufacturer of each product to be administered, to verify the recommended dose, formula, method and duration of administration, adverse effects and contraindications. It is the responsibility of the practitioner to take all appropriate safety precautions. Neither the publisher nor the author(s)/editor(s) assume any liability for any injury and/or damage to persons or property arising from or related to use of material in this book.

This book is sold on the understanding that the publisher is not engaged in providing professional medical services. If such advice or services are required, the services of a competent medical professional should be sought.

Every effort has been made where necessary to contact holders of copyright to obtain permission to reproduce copyright material. If any have been inadvertently overlooked, the publisher will be pleased to make the necessary arrangements at the first opportunity.

Inquiries for bulk sales may be solicited at: jaypee@jaypeebrothers.com

Molecular Pathology (PCRs & IHC)

First Edition: **2024**

ISBN: 978-93-5696-577-5

Preface

Molecular pathology truthfully took wings in the early 1990s when polymerase chain reaction (PCR) and immunohistochemistry (IHC) were in their nascent stages, which became its two main pillars.

Molecular genetics has been playing an increasingly important role in patient care and pathology practice. IHC is a valuable and practical tool employed by most pathologists on a regular basis.

Molecular pathology can be broadly defined as the testing of nucleic acids within a clinical context. The applications of molecular diagnostics span a range of human disorders, including hereditary, neoplastic, and infectious diseases. Molecular-based assays are used for specific purposes, including the following:

- Establishing the basis of an existing disorder (diagnostic testing)
- Determining the presence of a genetic condition when there are no obvious symptoms (predictive testing)
- Carrier testing
- Assessing a fetus for abnormalities (prenatal testing)
- Detecting cancer-causing gene mutations
- Selecting pharmacotherapy

The PCR is a method widely used to make millions to billions of copies of a specific DNA sample rapidly, allowing scientists to amplify a very small sample of DNA (or a part of it) sufficiently to enable detailed study. PCR was invented in 1983 by American biochemist Kary Mullis at Cetus Corporation. Mullis and biochemist Michael Smith, who had developed other essential ways of manipulating DNA, were jointly awarded the Nobel Prize in Chemistry in 1993.

The PCR is fundamental to many of the procedures used in genetic testing and research, including analysis of ancient samples of DNA and identification of infectious agents. Using PCR, copies of very small amounts of DNA sequences are exponentially amplified in a series of cycles of temperature changes. PCR is now a common and often indispensable technique used in medical laboratory research for a broad variety of applications including biomedical research and forensic science.

The book clearly outlines the basics of PCRs, history and the future is set to develop vis-à-vis this format as a diagnostic tool. The first five chapters take you into the world of PCRs—technology, hardware, and consumables. A small chapter is provided for you to grasp the technique in a jiffy.

The science that most histopathologists employ is IHC. But before one delves deep into the IHC protocols, one has to be perfect in histopathology techniques as this forms the basis of IHC itself. Both are lucidly presented in the last three chapters. Immunofluorescence (IF) and in situ hybridization (ISH) have not been forgotten as they too are components of molecular pathology.

Do take a peep inside. Happy reading!

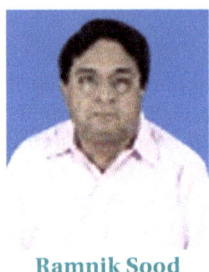

Ramnik Sood

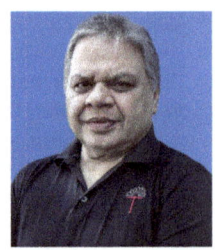

Deepak G Tripathi

Acknowledgments

We would like to thank the team of M/s Jaypee Brothers Medical Publishers (P) Ltd., New Delhi, India, Shri Jitendar P Vij (Group Chairman), Mr Ankit Vij (Managing Director), Mr MS Mani (Group President), Dr Madhu Choudhary (Director-Educational Publishing), Ms Pooja Bhandari [Director-Production (Books and Journals)], Mr Ajay Kumar Sharma [Deputy General Manager (Books and Journals)], Ms Sunita Katla (Executive Assistant to Group Chairman and Publishing Manager), Ms Samina Khan (Executive Assistant to Director-Educational Publishing) for their kind support.

We also acknowledge the help of Dr Upma Tomar (Development Editor), Mr Rajesh Sharma (Production Coordinator), Ms Seema Dogra (Cover Visualizer), Ms Neha (Cover Designer), Mr Kulwant Singh (Typesetter), and Mr Nitesh Jain (Graphic Designer), Mr Mithlesh Singh (Proofreader), and wish to thank all others of M/s Jaypee Brothers Medical Publishers (P) Ltd, New Delhi, without them this venture would not have been possible.

Contents

Chapter 1: Molecular Pathology — 1
- ❖ Digital Pathology *18*
- ❖ Molecular Pathology—The Future Ahead *20*

Chapter 2: PCRs-Technology, Techniques, History and Challenges — 22
- ❖ Brief History of Molecular Diagnostic Techniques *23*
- ❖ Molecular Diagnostic Techniques *24*
- ❖ Polymerase Chain Reaction *34*
- ❖ Real Time PCR and RT PCR *36*
- ❖ PCR Components *37*
- ❖ Real-time PCR Analysis and Troubleshooting *45*
- ❖ List of Troubleshooting Graphs *62*
- ❖ Application of Molecular Diagnostics *73*
- ❖ Evolution of PCR *75*
- ❖ Journey of RT PCR *80*
- ❖ Current Challenges *81*

Chapter 3: Polymerase Chain Reaction in Clinical Diagnosis (Recapitulation in Brief) — 85
- ❖ Evolution of PCRs *85*
- ❖ Applications of PCR *97*
- ❖ Advantages of PCR over Conventional Techniques *97*
- ❖ Limitations/Difficulties *98*

Chapter 4: Practical Aspects/Actual Working on Systems Amplichain™ 100

- ❖ Current Challenge in Performing Real-time PCR System *100*
- ❖ What is the Need? *102*
- ❖ Objective and Purpose *103*
- ❖ Introduction of Amplichain Instrument and Reagent *103*

Chapter 5: Commercially Available–Kits of an Open System 123
Innovative Ideas Simplifying Molecular Diagnostics 123
- ❖ Amplichain *123*

Amplichain 125
- ❖ Simplifying Molecular Diagnostics *125*
- ❖ Universal Nucleic Acid Extraction Kit *126*
- ❖ Simplifying Molecular Diagnostics *127*

Amplichain® Universal (Magnetic Bead Method) 130
- ❖ Intended Use *130*

Amplichain Chikungunya 140
- ❖ Description *140*
- ❖ Assay Performance *155*

Any parameter PCR Testing Follows the Same Procedural Protocols Barring a Few Reagent Changes 160
- ❖ Available Parameters Commercially World Over *160*

Chapter 6: Histopathology (Prelude to Immunohistochemistry) 163
- ❖ Tissue Fixation and Gross Examination *165*
- ❖ Tissue Processing and Embedding *192*
- ❖ Staining Techniques *238*

Chapter 7: Immunohistochemistry 263
- ❖ Common Hitches Observed at End Result of the Immunohistochemistry *327*

- Application of Immunohistochemistry *328*
- Immunofluorescence Technique (IF) *332*
- In Situ Hybridization (ISH) *336*

Annexures 341
- Annexure I *341*
- Annexure II *342*

Index *345*

CHAPTER 1

Molecular Pathology

BACKGROUND

If one compares the role of pathology in medicine to a tree, it gets obvious that the roots are the foundations, basic science, and the branches are different clinical specialties **(Fig. 1.1)**, molecular pathology is based on the principles, techniques, and tools of molecular biology **(Fig. 1.2)** as they are applied to diagnostic medicine in the clinical laboratory. The field of molecular pathology is "so rapidly changing that you can't just focus on one thing for the future. The diversification, the perception of transcending sequencing; it is evidently going beyond genomics. Though Informatics helps us with the ever-increasing complexity in molecular data, there is a crying need to embrace new technology and products to exploit what's newly available. As molecular biology methods are being used to elucidate the genetic and molecular basis of many diseases, such discoveries have ultimately led to the emergence of predictive molecular pathology. In the current situation, where our country and the world faces a Covid-19 pandemic, the shining beacon that helped turn the tide on this pandemic was the ability of molecular diagnostic testing, by laboratories worldwide. The practice of molecular pathology

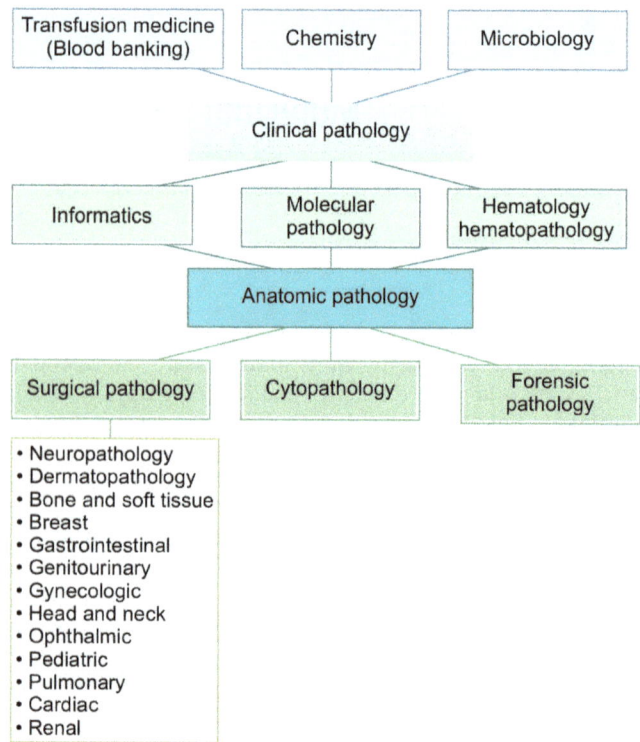

Fig. 1.1: Different clinical specialties of molecular pathology.

has been and continues to be dependent upon new and robust molecular diagnostic technologies to interrogate DNA and/or RNA sequences for detection of sequence variants associated with a particular diagnosis, prognosis, or therapeutic response.

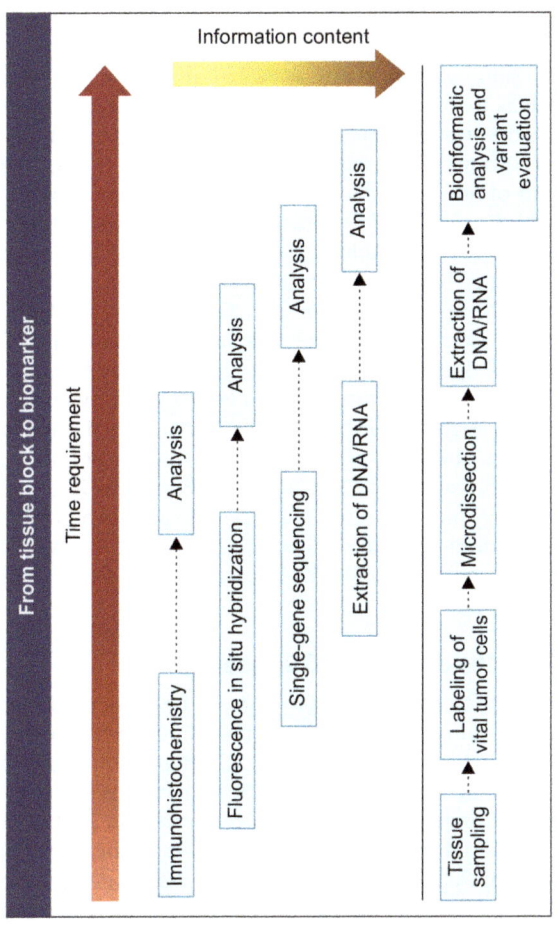

Fig. 1.2: Techniques of molecular pathology.

INTRODUCTION

Newer developments are taking place daily in the field of molecular pathology as the need for genetic disease, hematologic disease, infectious disease, pharmacogenomic, solid tumor, and identity testing continues to increase. The rapid pace of change due to the advent of new technology, ongoing discovery of the nature of different diseases, and the development of new treatments all mean that molecular pathology is in a flux of continuous evolution. As technologies become more robust, faster, and cheaper, the adoption of the not-so-common tests will also increase. Hence, it is clear why research in molecular pathology is the catalyst for a sea change in which pathologists, clinicians, and key stakeholders from across the care continuum need to be deeply involved with the common goal of improving molecular diagnostics for today and for the establishing predictive molecular pathology as the cornerstone of the future. Only by assimilating new information and technology into pathology practices can patient outcomes be improved continuously and consistently. This is visibly evident from the irrefutable contribution of molecular pathology to various facets of science.

Molecular Pathology and ONCO Diagnostics

Molecular pathology is evolving to address the challenge of cancer and improve cancer diagnostics/therapies. It is well known that cancer is caused by a combination of inherited and progressively acquired genetic mutations in specific cells that give rise to the tumor. Examining the tumor's genetic material can lead to a very complex yet highly specific diagnosis. Based on the detection of these point molecular alterations, with a clear oncogenic role, treatments have been developed to block the activation of mutated, amplified proteins or product of translocations by specific drugs. It is only with molecular pathology at the molecular components of the cells, like DNA and RNA, and other cellular constituents such as proteins, that many further divisions of these types can be identified. A diagnosis based on the genetic or molecular profile of the tumor indicates which targeted therapies are likely to provide better efficacy, now and in the future when new targeted therapies are available. Finding the optimal treatment for a patient based on an individualized diagnosis is a move away from what has been referred to as the 'trial-and-error' approach of prescribing. This approach also has the potential to improve patient quality of life by reducing their experience of adverse events by choosing a therapy suited to the patient's tumor profile and importantly, targeted therapies have been shown to enable patients to live longer when compared with nontargeted therapies in a range of cancers. Hence, the identification of patients with therapeutic molecular targets in their tumors is currently a standard of care. Notwithstanding that, the initial morphological diagnosis and the eventual tumor classification by immunohistochemistry (IHC), as well as the acquisition, handling and processing of tumor tissue play a pivotal role. As this aspect of molecular pathology grows more complex and specialized, it is not easy for physicians and healthcare leaders to keep up-to-date with the changes—particularly when contact time with pathologists is limited. For patients, pathology can just be a report, but for the clinicians involved with the therapies, improved understanding and collaboration in molecular pathology is a must, to capitalize on the ever-evolving sciences that bring about targeted therapies. As cancer diagnoses get more complex, requiring integration of multiple types of testing, regular interactions between the pathologist and the treating physician about the implications of diagnosis gets priceless because the pathologist brings perspectives that others do not have. If molecular pathology reveals that a lung cancer patient, for example, has a mutation of the epidermal growth factor receptor (EGFR) gene, then treatment with a targeted EGFR-inhibitor therapy has been shown to improve survival. Various studies of malignant tumors in infants have found gene fusions to be present in relatively rare tumor subtypes. With the discussions around gene fusions including those involving neurotrophic receptor tyrosine kinase (NTRK), anaplastic lymphoma kinase (ALK) and the proto-oncogene 1, receptor tyrosine kinase (ROS1); the therapeutic value of targeting them is now being recognized. However, the combination of less invasive techniques that provide very small samples to carry out an increasing number of determinations is controversial, since it does not allow to increase the amount of tumor cells. Consequently, more sensitive and specific molecular determinations are required.

Molecular Pathology and Next-generation Sequencing

Next-generation sequencing (NGS) technique is a useful and novel tool for the study of molecular profile from DNA/RNA and the treatment of cancer patients has evolved with the addition of new massive sequencing technologies, in this decade. Tumor heterogeneity and the addition of new molecular targets have become a challenge that needs a multidisciplinary approach and learning, with the study of the molecular profile of the tumor at the genomic (DNA), transcriptomic (RNA) or protein (protein) level. NGS can be used to sequence either whole genomes or specific genomic areas of interest, including all 22,000 coding genes—the whole-genome sequencing (WGS), the whole exome sequencing (WES)—a genomic technique for sequencing all of the protein-coding regions of genes in a genome, known as the exome; or small numbers of individual genes (NGS panels). Although capillary-based cancer sequencing has been ongoing for over a decade; these investigations had been restricted to relatively few samples and small numbers of candidate genes. But, over the last years, NGS has evolved and transitioned as an interesting, massive parallel sequencing platform at various molecular pathology routine laboratories for the simultaneous analysis of multiple genes with low input material. To do the library using amplicon methods, it is only necessary to obtain 10 ng of DNA just from the tumor, and 10 ng of RNA, which is feasible, even from small samples, fixed in formalin and included in paraffin. But laboratories working with formalin-fixed paraffin embedded (FFPE) material and high sample throughput largely require high-quality DNA obtained from automated DNA extraction systems. Parallel sequencing requires target enrichment, which is a pre-sequencing step that only allows part of a whole-genome be sequenced, or regions of interest, without sequencing the entire genome of a sample. The two most commonly used techniques for NGS target enrichment are capture hybridization and amplicon-based (multiplex PCR). The extension/ligation occurs between hybrid probes which determines a uniquely tagged amplicon library ready for cluster generation and sequencing. The spectrum of DNA variation in a human genome comprises:

- Small base changes (substitutions)
- Insertions and deletions of DNA
- Large genomic deletions of exons or whole genes, and
- Rearrangements, such as inversions and translocations.

Considering the WGS method in the same fresh and FFPE samples, hybrid capture sequencing showed higher sensitivity compared to amplicon sequencing, while maintaining 100% specificity using Sanger sequencing as a validation method. Traditional Sanger sequencing focuses on the discovery of substitutions and small insertions and deletions. Amplicon method has higher target rates. Hybridization capture-based approaches demonstrated that many of them could be false positives or negatives. These results reveal advantages and disadvantages of both methods. On occasions, an extremely sensitive method is not worth using given its clinical implications.

Molecular Pathology and Personalized Medicine

To understand which personalized medicine strategy or therapeutic options will be effective, a different approach to diagnostics is needed and this is where molecular pathology plays a vital role without which, personalized medicine would not be possible. Personalized medicine allows the identification of patients that can benefit from targeted therapies, since the molecular characteristics of the diseases can be identified. Over the last decade, new drugs have been incorporated into the treatment, including the development of immunotherapy and treatment against specific molecular targets. In particular, personalized medicine has started a revolution in cancer care. For many patients, it is proving to be utterly transformative. The basic premise of cancer genomics is that cancer is caused by somatically acquired mutations and is therefore a disease of the genome. This has contributed to the study of tumor biology with an accurate and highly covered diagnostic method that allows the selection of those patients likely to benefit most from target-specific targeted therapies. By taking into account a patient's genetic and molecular profile, their treatment can be tailored to the individual, and it is commonly far more effective, improving quality of life and helping patients to live longer. Thus, patients can receive specific treatments according to the biology of their tumor, turning oncology into a tool for personalized medicine. In order to do so, the development of new DNA/RNA sequencing technologies is required, as well as the development of specific antibodies identifying mutated or altered proteins, and the design of new in situ hybridization techniques. The latter has enabled the selection via genetic biomarkers of patients, who can benefit from therapies targeted against specific molecular alterations. The prevalence of molecular alterations with targeted treatment may vary according to different variables, such as the region of the world, race and gender. About 86% of tumors have molecular alterations that can potentially be treatable with approved or developing drugs, of which approximately 30% have clinically available drugs. The distribution of these alterations in patients with metastatic disease varies compares to those observed in resected tumors at earlier stages. Even as cancer numbers rise, patients are missing out on molecular testing and on subsequent targeted therapy. These are challenges which must be addressed if the potential of personalized medicine due to molecular pathology is to be unlocked.

Molecular Pathology and Cancers—Classical Relevant Instance

Molecular pathology is increasingly being used for typing of neoplasms, risk assessment and directing cancer treatment. Nowhere are the recent developments in such molecular stratification more evident than in breast and endometrial carcinoma. Endometrial carcinoma (EC) is the most common gynecological malignancy in the developed world with increasing annual incidence and mortality rates in North America. Similar to the progress made in breast cancer, where subtyping integrates molecular information for stratification, molecular subtyping of EC has emerged as a priority in the gynecological oncology sphere. In 2013, the Cancer Genome Atlas (TCGA) published a comprehensive genomic analysis of EC **(Figs. 1.3A to D)** (endometrioid, serous and mixed histotypes, n = 373). The TCGA described four prognostically distinct groups, **(Fig. 1.1)**

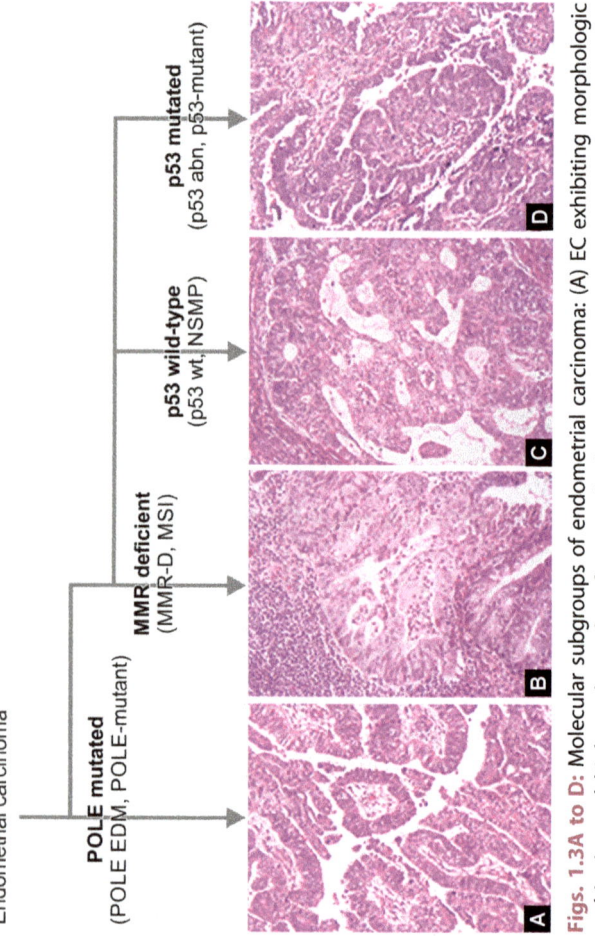

Figs. 1.3A to D: Molecular subgroups of endometrial carcinoma: (A) EC exhibiting morphologic ambiguity and high-grade nuclear features, harboring a POLE exonuclease domain mutation; (B) EC showing dense peritumoral lymphocytic inflammation, harboring deficient of mismatch repair proteins; (C) EC with low-grade features, exhibiting no specific mutation profile (NSMP, p53 wild-type); (D) EC with serous morphology, harboring a TP53 mutation.

characterized by tumor mutational burden and somatic copy number alterations:

Endometrial carcinomas (EC) represent four different molecular subgroups:
1. Ultramutated EC with DNA polymerase epsilon (POLE) mutations in the exonuclease domain (POLE EDM),
2. Hypermutated EC with microsatellite instability (MSI),
3. Low mutation rate EC with low frequency of DNA copy-number alterations (CN-L), and
4. Low mutation rate EC but with high-frequency of DNA copy-number alterations (CNeH).

In terms of somatic mutations:
- Ultramutated EC were enriched in ARID1A (>70%), FBXW7 (>80%), KRAS (>50%) and PI3K pathway (>70%) mutations,
- Hypermutated EC = the highest RPL22 (>40%),
- CN-L EC = the highest CTNNBI (>50%), and
- CN-HEC = highest TP53 (>90%) and lowest frequency of PTEN (<10%) mutations.

The TCGA also revealed that molecularly distinct ECs exhibited overlapping histologic features, as well as vice versa, that biologically similar EC can have varied morphologic appearances. This served as a catalyst for the development of a pragmatic molecular-based classification strategy that could be adopted in everyday practice. Emergence of pragmatic risk classifiers for EC is the outcome. Using immunohistochemistry (IHC), targeted sequencing and MSI testing, two different molecular classification schemes emerged. Both classifiers produced results that emulated the four TCGA based molecular subtypes.

ProMisE, developed by Talhouk et al. in 2015 recapitulated the 4 TGCA risk groups by using IHC for p53 and mismatch repair (MMR) proteins, together with sequencing for POLE exonuclease

domain mutations (EDM). In the ProMisE classification system, four groups, serving as corollaries to the TGCA groups **(Fig. 1.2)** described above, were:
1. POLE EDM
2. MMR-D
3. p53 wt
4. p53 abn.

This iterative classifier has been confirmed in various studies across multiple cohorts.

The other, by Stelloo et al. was based on a comprehensive molecular analysis of high risk EC from PORTEC (post operative radiation therapy in endometrial carcinoma). They performed MSI testing, targeted mutational testing (including POLE) and IHC (including p53). **(Table 1.1)**. Their results independently confirmed the four prognostic groups. Excellent concordance in molecular subtyping between biopsy and hysterectomy specimens has been independently demonstrated and the benefits for upfront triaging includes improved accuracy of IHC interpretation due to improved fixation in biopsy specimens and the provision of prognostic and predictive information for subsequent treatment planning.

Based on these observations, it is now evident that molecular subtyping in EC is poised to become 'standard of care' in the diagnosis of ECC. Pragmatic molecular classifiers for EC based of the TCGA have been developed, which strategize EC into four groups—POLE mutated, MMR-D/MSI, p53 mutated and p53 wild type (no specific mutation profile). These four molecular subgroups confer clinical and prognostic information for tailored treatment strategies. Multiple classifier cases are still defined by their truncal molecular subtype. EC with subclonal MMR loss should undergo testing for MLH1 hypermethylation testing, as the majority are due to epigenetic MLH1 gene silencing. EC with subclonal

Table 1.1: Molecular subtypes of endometrial carcinoma.

	Major molecular subtypes of endometrial carcinoma			
	POLE EDM	**MMR-D**	**p53 wt**	**p53 abn**
Alternate names	Ultramutated POLE-mut	Hypermutated MMRd	Copy number low NSMP	Copy number high p53-mut
Salient molecular alterations	Mutation in POLE exonuclease domain • High mutational burden (>100 mutations/Mb) • Low copy number alterations • Mutations in PI3K pathway	Microsatellite instability high. • Deficiency in mismatch repair proteins • Intermediate mutational burden • Low copy number alterations	TP53 wild type • Low mutational burden (<10/Mb) • High copy number alterations Mutations in PI3K and Wnt/β-catenin pathways	TP53 mutated • Low mutational burden (<10/Mb) • Low copy number alterations • Rare mutations in ERBB2 and BRCA
Proportion	5%	25%	45%	25%
Clinical and prognostic features	Age ~ 50–60 Pre/postmenopausal • Low BMI • Early stage and excellent outcomes	Age ~60 Perimenopausal High BMI Intermediate outcomes	Age ~ 60 • Perimenopausal • High BMI • Intermediate outcomes	Age ~ 70 • Postmenopausal • Low BMI • High-stage and poor outcomes

Major molecular subtypes of endometrial carcinoma

	POLE EDM	MMR-D	p53 wt	p53 abn
Histologic features	• Mix of low-grade and high grade endometrioid histology • Ambiguous morphology, peri/intratumoral lymphocytes • Can be associated with subclonal p53 patterns	• Mix of low-grade and high grade endometrioid histology • Ambiguous morphology, peri/intratumoral lymphocytes substantial lymphovascular invasion • Can be associated with subclonal p53 and MMR IHC patterns	• Mostly low-grade endometrioid histology • Tend to express ER and PR	• Mostly serous histology • Destructive growth patterns and lymphovascular invasion
Treatment implications	Immune checkpoint inhibition	Immune checkpoint inhibition referral to hereditary cancer program for suspected lynch syndrome	• Hormonal management • Fertility sparing management may be considered	Possible role for HER2 and PARP inhibitors

p53 IHC should prompt evaluation by MMR IHC and POLE mutation testing to achieve accurate risk stratification.

Molecular Pathology and Nucleic Acid Testing Automation

Many molecular diagnostic tests require nucleic acid extraction, an analytical procedure such as polymerase chain reaction (PCR) or sequencing, and then data analysis and reporting. Advances in molecular pathology has enabled this three-step process to be combined into the workflow of a single test. Automating this workflow improves patient safety by reducing sample test time or misidentification errors and benefits the patient by reducing the time on diagnostic processes, leading to quicker interventions and faster turnaround time. The field of molecular diagnostics has begun to evolve rapidly with the evolution of newer diseases periodically like Bird flu, H1N1, Ebola, Nipah virus, Zika, etc., with the need for more molecular-based tests far outweighing the commercial and financial interests. So, even though test volumes may be relatively low compared to common clinical laboratory tests, newer primers/probes targeting genes of clinical interest for emerging diseases are undergoing a boom. In this context, PCR variations merit attention like polymorphisms. Polymorphisms are inherited differences found among the individuals in a population at a frequency >1% of that population. The term "polymorphism" is not synonymous with the term "mutation" which is used for germline variations that are pathogenic and found less frequently in a population or are nongermline changes in a tumor cell (somatic mutations). In the case of restriction fragment length polymorphisms (RFLP), DNA sequence differences alter RE recognition sites, manifested either as obliteration or creation of a restriction site. With obliteration of a RE site, the DNA of individuals with an RFLP exhibits a larger restriction fragment of DNA than those without the polymorphism.

With creation of a new RE site, RE digestion results in two smaller fragments relative to the individual without the polymorphism. In either case, the polymorphism is detectable by creation of a new restriction fragment pattern, that is, a restriction fragment length polymorphism. In PCR-RFLP, the PCR products are digested by one or a combination of REs and electrophoresed to detect polymorphisms or mutations which are seen as changes in the DNA fragment sizes reflected by changes in the band pattern on the gel (or chromatogram). Examples of applications of PCR-RFLP analysis:

* Detection of sickle-cell hemoglobin (HbS) gene mutation
* Detection of the MnlI restriction enzyme polymorphism created by the Factor V Leiden mutation

Some DNA sequence variants create or abolish RE recognition sites and can easily be detected by PCRRFLP. Unfortunately, most variants do not alter a RE recognition site. In restriction-site generating PCR (RG-PCR) (and a related research technique called PCR-mediated site directed mutagenesis [PSDM]), an artificial RE recognition site is generated during PCR using a specially designed PCR primer. The primer contains a base mismatch to the template DNA adjacent to the variable base of the variant that creates a RE recognition site in the PCR product. The mismatched base in the primer is located near or at the 3' end of the primer, which is near or adjacent to the variable base of the variant, and together they create a novel restriction site within either the variant or non-variant amplicon. The presence or absence of the RE recognition site is determined from the pattern of digested PCR product fragments by gel electrophoresis. Examples of Applications of RG-PCR:

* Identification of mutations in the CTFR gene in cystic fibrosis
* Identification of mutations in the ATM gene in ataxia–telangiectasis

Multiplex PCR is a technique used for amplification of several discrete genetic loci with multiple PCR primer pairs in a single reaction. Multiplex PCR simultaneously answers several related questions about a specimen without the need for multiple individual PCR reactions. Multiplex PCR is commonly used for verification that amplifiable nucleic acid is present in the sample, for example, amplification of a housekeeping gene in addition to the gene sequence(s) of interest, and to check for the presence of PCR inhibitors that can prevent amplification of target nucleic acid. Another method for a multiplexed assay is single nucleotide extension (SNE) or single base extension (SBE). SNE and SBE can be considered sequencing, but of just one base. Examples of Applications of SNE:

* Analysis of common mutations in GALT for galactosemia
* Analysis of common mutations in BTD for biotinidase deficiency
* Analysis of multiple mutations in the CFTR gene for cystic fibrosis

Nested PCR involves checking for two pairs of PCR primers with one set internal to the other (nested) are used to sequentially amplify a single locus. The first pair is used to amplify the locus as in any PCR assay. A dilution of the first PCR reaction then is amplified with the nested primers. Alternatively, seminested PCR is performed using one of the original PCR primers and one new internal primer in a second round of amplification. Both nested and semi-nested PCR generate a second PCR product that is shorter than the first one. The logic behind this strategy is that if the wrong locus was amplified incorrectly or non-specifically, the probability is very low that it would be amplified a second time by a second pair of primers. Thus, nested PCR enhances specificity while also increasing sensitivity. The problem with nested PCR is the high risk of amplicon contamination when the first-round PCR products are used to set up the second round of PCR with the nested primers. For this reason, many clinical laboratories do not use nested PCR procedures.

It is worth mentioning that laboratory developed tests (LDTs), also commonly referred to as "homebrew" assays have grown across the world representing the "freedom to operate" and the need to keep up with the pace of new molecular discoveries so as to rapidly deliver those to clinical practice. But the problem with such tests is that without proper regulatory validation, it veers towards doubtful reliability due to lack of appropriate positive samples and control materials. In this context, the evolution of globally certified and accepted Truenat® from India is indeed a revolutionary accessory to all molecular pathologists. With minimal intervention and capabilities to function smoothly in resource limited settings, introductions like these will transform molecular pathology testing across the world and convert a once rare test into a daily routine.

DIGITAL PATHOLOGY

The future of pathology will be a balanced synthesis of human and machine, enabling delivery of healthcare that is timely, appropriate, and effective. Recent advances in whole slide imaging (WSI) have catalyzed clinical deployment of digital pathology (DP) hardware and software at sites across the globe, allowing pathologists to make primary diagnoses on the digital microscope, and laying the foundations for the future implementation of AI tools in clinical pathology to assist in diagnosis and disease management. Digital pathology [DP] is defined as a pathological diagnosis transmitted over a distance, together with specific digital images of micro- and macroscopic preparations, clinical data, and information on cases sent to a pathologist via a data link. DP makes archiving and accessing images quicker and easier, and archives of high-resolution diagnostic images have the potential to provide real world training datasets that can be used to create AI apps. For example, an app might pre-screen lymph node tissue to detect regions suspicious for tumor metastasis. Ideally, such apps fit into the workflow that is enabled by DP, allowing the app to become an important part of the diagnostic process. Some apps of this type have already been developed, executing tumor detection, diagnosis, grading as well as prognostic and predictive tasks. Microscopic analyses have shifted from FOV (static) images to WSI and from one to multiple markers (multiplexing), often even using many colors (multispectral imaging). Ai based algorithms offer better accuracy, because they provide more precise and even continuous quantitative measurements compared with humans. Using image algorithms also permits standardization due to more reproducible results, especially for intermediate scoring categories and complex scoring systems . The benefits of DP and AI must be relevant to the patient's experience of their healthcare and their health outcomes. Many aspects of DP and AI also benefit the patient as time saved on diagnostic processes can lead to quicker interventions and faster turnaround time. DP has the capacity to improve patient safety by reducing sample and test result misidentification errors that can arise when transferring patient information from one medium to another. AI could support clinical decisions by rapidly providing an accurate contribution to the diagnostic and prognostic process. But there is much more to come. With the development of deep learning, AI is being used to carry out more complex tasks in histology, image recognition and classification. In deep learning, the systems created behave much more like the human brain, with layers of 'neural' (computational) networks that can develop their own algorithms without the need for algorithms to be inputted beforehand. Although there are questions around the regulatory approval of AI apps as well as the development and production costs to prevent DP and AI from replacing the pathologist completely, there are other reasons why the future will not be an AI-only zone, that excludes the pathologist. The responsibility for making the crucial decisions which diagnose a patient and monitor their response to treatment or recurrence of disease are best carried out by machine and human working together. Why is this so? Addition of human insight and creative thought to provide a fully rounded clinical opinion for each patient is needed to take into account all elements of a patient's life and arrive at a diagnosis, something that an AI pathology app cannot.

MOLECULAR PATHOLOGY—THE FUTURE AHEAD

All specialties of medicine perceive molecular pathology and molecular diagnostics as the future because with the amount of data available and analyzed currently, molecular pathology is entrenching itself firmly as the fulcrum of the future in the very middle of changing paradigms on therapies. As this is going to be even more challenging in the future, we need to be ready for whatever changes come our way. In fact, it is said that molecular pathology generates 75% of the data that determines 75% of the downstream action in the medical management of patients. Despite traditional histopathology still providing essential information for cancer diagnosis on cancer type and grade, molecular pathology by providing a greater level of detail about each patient's tumor brings opportunities for better advantages. Molecular pathology is essential to the provision of personalized medicine, now and more so in the future. The molecular profile is nowadays an essential additional tool for pathology practice, which invariably enables the in-depth study of molecular alterations in patients thus optimizing molecular diagnosis and selecting patients to receive novel treatments, targeted against specific molecular targets for the clinical benefit of patients, through a multidisciplinary approach and learning. If this opportunity to provide accurate, in-depth diagnosis at the very beginning of each patient's treatment journey is not utilized effectively, the treatment outcomes for patients may be significantly impaired, and the service of healing may suffer. The amount and type of data is expanding and changing dramatically with the greater adoption of personalized medicine. Although, in recent times, there is a huge increase in people coming in to work in AI, we're still some way off from this integrated routinely. With AI/ML in the future, how we teach and test will be key. When we initially compared the efficiency and productivity of pathologists with AI/ML, it was always people who came out as winners, but now we're seeing a shift with AI/ML starting to win more. As automation becomes a larger part of many clinical labs, the role of artificial intelligence (AI)/ machine learning (ML) is expected to impact molecular pathology as well. Four key words that can describe the future of molecular pathology are: collaboration, communication, involvement, and evolution with the key demands being met by potentially faster and more accurate technologies. Molecular imaging is the most promising field showing the potential to achieve the integration of a noninvasive, safe, and fast examination method into routine clinical practice. This integration would result in a new pattern of pathological practice—the concept of "transpathology", whereby pathological lesions could be visualized to transparentize tissue and not only better present the underlying pathophysiological information, but also better facilitate the translational processes from the bench to the bedside.

CHAPTER 2

PCRs-Technology, Techniques, History and Challenges

INTRODUCTION

The application of nucleic acid-based testing to disease diagnosis and therapy with high accuracy and reduced cost offers revolutionary progress in human and animal genomics and this has improved the fundamentals of medicine and treatment regime.

Previously and in recent past the analysis of deoxyribonucleic acid (DNA) by scientists was difficult due to small structure of nucleic acid. Also, the examination of nucleotides sequences that formed the genetic material of organism was only possible indirectly through protein or ribonucleic acid (RNA) sequencing or by genetic analysis. However, other approaches involving the direct analysis of DNA, isolation of specific regions of genomes and manipulation of genes in genetic engineering and recombinant DNA technology have been developed.

Molecular biology is the molecular basis of biological activity between biomolecules in the various cellular systems of the body. Biological activities in the body include biosynthesis of DNA, RNA and proteins, and the interactions between these molecules and the regulations of their interactions.

Molecular diagnostics on the other hand are collections of techniques used in the analysis of biological markers in the genome and proteome by applying molecular biology to medical testing. These techniques have been reported to be vital in the diagnosis of inherited genetic diseases such as cystic fibrosis and hemochromatosis, infectious diseases, oncology, leukocyte antigen typing (HLA).

Molecular diagnostics therefore provides relevant preliminary information for the successful application of gene therapy, biologic response modifiers, the assessment of disease prognosis and therapy response as well as detection of minimal residual disease. Hence, this technical series provides a summary of the history, various types and applications of commonly utilized molecular diagnostic techniques in biological sciences.

BRIEF HISTORY OF MOLECULAR DIAGNOSTIC TECHNIQUES

The field of molecular biology and its clinical application grown in the late twentieth century. In 1980, prenatal genetic test for thalassemia was suggested and this test relied on restriction enzymes (endonuclease such as Bam HI) that cut DNA.

This test allowed for the recognition of specific short sequences, created by different lengths of DNA strands dependent on the allele (variant form of the gene). In the 1980s, phrases used in the names of companies involved in developing these techniques included Molecular Diagnostics Incorporated, Bethesda Research Laboratories Molecular Diagnostics etc. In the 1990s, a distinct field of molecular and genomic laboratory medicine was developed following the identification of newly discovered genes and new techniques for DNA sequencing.

In 1995, the Association for Molecular Pathology (AMP) was formed to follow up on the new discoveries which led to establishment of The Journal of Medical Diagnostics in 1999. The Expert Reviews in The Journal of Medical Diagnostics was launched in by Informa Healthcare. Later in 2002, information regarding recurrence of one-letter genetic differences (the single nucleotide polymorphisms) in human population as well as their relationship with the disease was accumulated and published.

In 2012, molecular diagnostic techniques for thalassemia use genetic hybridization tests to identify the specific single nucleotide polymorphism causing an individual's disease. However, the importance of commercial application of molecular diagnostics has created debate about patenting of the genetic discoveries at its heart. In 1998, the European Union's Directive 98/44/EC clarified that patents on DNA sequences were allowable. In 2010 in the US, AMP sued Myriad Genetics to challenge the latter's patents regarding two genes, BRCA1and BRCA2, which are associated with breast cancer. In 2013, the U.S. Supreme Court partially agreed, ruling that a naturally occurring gene sequence could not be patented. With advancement in molecular diagnostics, the detection of specific nucleotide sequences in DNA and RNA related or unrelated to disease has been made possible. These nucleotide sequences may be due to changes such as gene rearrangements, insertion and deletion.

This therefore has led to the efficiency, accuracy and rapid growth in diagnostic with accentuation of personalized therapy.

MOLECULAR DIAGNOSTIC TECHNIQUES

Molecular Cloning

In molecular biology, molecular cloning has been used as a basic tool to highlight the functions of proteins. In this technique, DNA coding for a protein of interest is cloned (using PCR and/or restriction enzymes) into a plasmid (known as an expression vector).

This plasmid can be inserted into either bacterial or animal cells. Introducing DNA into bacterial cells can be done by transformation (via uptake of naked DNA), conjugation (via cell-cell contact) or by transduction (via viral vector) **(Fig. 2.1)**.

Introducing DNA into eukaryotic cells, such as animal cells, by physical or chemical means is called transfection. Several transfection techniques are available, and these include calcium phosphate transfection, electroporation, microinjection and liposome transfection. DNA can also be introduced into eukaryotic cells using viruses or bacteria *(Agrobacterium tumefaciens)* as carriers; the latter is sometimes called bactofection.

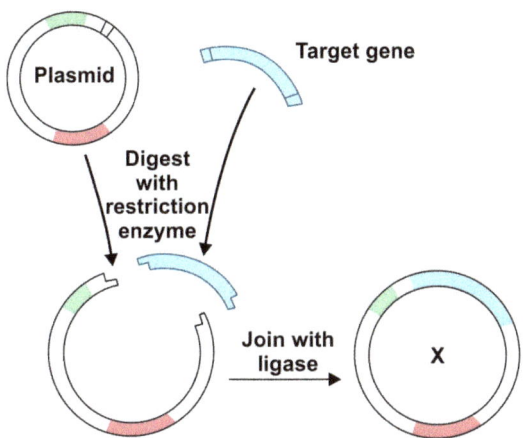

Fig. 2.1: Molecular cloning by plasmids.

In signaling factors, are available to help express the protein of interest at high levels molecular cloning, a variety of systems including inducible promoters and specific cell. Large quantities of a protein can then be extracted from the bacterial or eukaryotic cell.

Macromolecule Blotting and Probing

"**Blotting,**" is a term that refers to the process of detecting the presence and quantity of DNA, RNA, or protein in cells. The blotting and probing techniques were first described by Edwin Southern (1973) for the hybridization of blotted DNA. In 1984, Patricia Thomas developed the RNA blot and this became known as the northern blot. Further modifications and combinations of these protocols gave rise to other techniques such as south westerns (protein-DNA hybridizations), north westerns (to detect protein-RNA interactions) and far western (protein-protein interactions), as reported in literature.

Northern Blotting

In the northern blotting, **(Fig. 2.2)** the structure and quantity of RNA are emphasized in relation to their expression patterns among different samples of RNA. It is one of the most basic tools for determining the time, levels and conditions certain genes are expressed in living tissues. The protocol involves using a combination of denaturing RNA gel electrophoresis and a blot. In this technique, RNAs are separated based on size. The separated RNAs are then transferred to a membrane probed with a labeled complement of a sequence of interest. The results visualized in the establishment of bands represent the sizes of the RNA detected while the intensity of these bands is related to the amount of the target RNA in the samples analyzed. The procedure is commonly used to study when and how much gene expression is occurring by measuring the quantity of RNAs present in different samples.

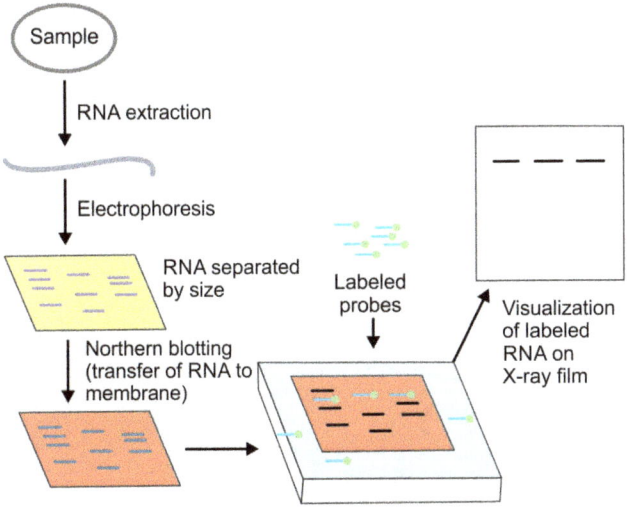

Fig. 2.2: Northern blotting.

The major disadvantages of the northern blot technique were its poor sensitivity and high time consumption due to the use of the traditional DNA oligonucleotide probes. These have been overcome by adoption of an improvised protocol of miRNA analysis involving RNA extraction polyacrylamide gel electrophoresis with northern blotting, and the detection of locked nucleic acid (LNA)-modified oligonucleotide probes by hybridization.

Western Blotting

In western blotting, **(Fig. 2.3)** the detection of proteins is first carried out followed by separation based on size and molecular weight using a thin gel sandwiched between two glass plates. This technique is referred to as sodium dodecyl sulphate polyacrylamide gel electrophoresis (SDS-PAGE).

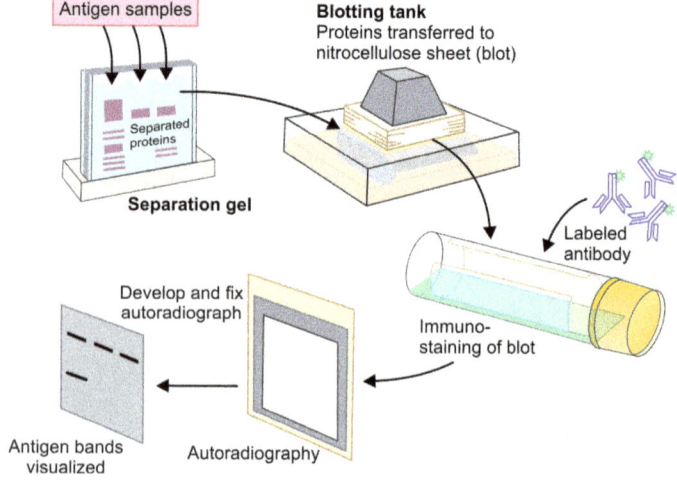

Fig. 2.3: Western blotting.

The proteins in the gel are then transferred to a support membrane probed with solutions of enzymes-labeled antibodies. These support membranes include polyvinylidene fluoride (PVDF), nitrocellulose, nylon etc. The specificity of antibodies-protein binding is visualized by a colored product (chemiluminescence) or autoradiography. However, the use of western blotting techniques allows for not only detection but also quantitative analysis.

Gel Electrophoresis

Gel electrophoresis is one of the basic tools of molecular biology. The term "electrophoresis" was originally meant to refer to the migration of charged molecular particles in an electrical field, especially across a membrane. However, the migration of lower molecular weight substances in stabilized media such as gels and powders has been referred to as "ionophoresis". The basic principle is that by means of an electric field and size, DNA, RNA, and proteins can all be separated. In agarose gel electrophoresis, DNA and RNA are separated based on size by running the substances through an electrically charged agarose gel.

Fluorescent in situ Hybridization

Fluorescent in situ hybridization (FISH) **(Fig. 2.4)** was developed by biomedical researchers in the 1980's and is based on the use of fluorescence-labelled oligonucleotide probes that specifically attach to their complementary DNA sequence target on the genome and the region is labelled with fluorescence color (e.g., Texas red, FITCI green, acridine orange). The labeled region can then be visualized under a fluorescence microscope. There are three types of probes in wide use:

1. **Painting probes:** Through the attaching of the painting probe to overlapping sequences on target chromosome (e.g., chromosome 17), the chromosome is identified as "painting" based on the chosen fluorescence color.
2. Centromeric probes that identify the centromeric region of a specific chromosome and thus help in enumerating the number of copies of that chromosome even in a nondividing cell interphase state [1982].

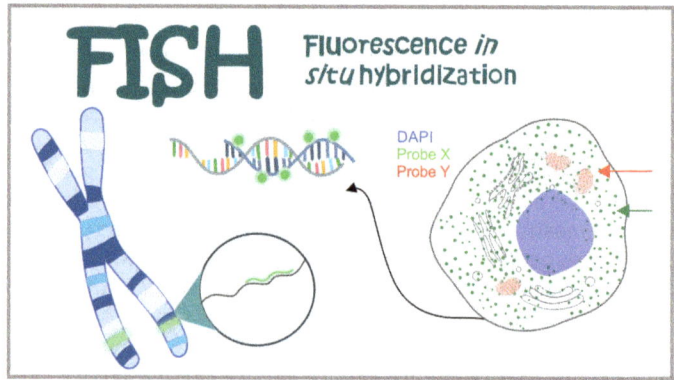

Fig. 2.4: Fluorescent in situ hybridization (FISH).

3. Allele-specific probes that adhere to a specific target allele sequence such as the p53 tumor suppressor gene or the HER2/neu oncogene.

FISH offers great advantages over conventional cytogenetics in the study of chromosomal deletions and translocations, and gene amplifications. Conventional cytogenetics requires a time-consuming cell culture step and can be performed only with fresh tissue samples. FISH is fast and sensitive and could be used as a complementary tool in genetic diagnostics as it can be performed on cells in dividing (metaphase) and resting (interphase) stages, fresh frozen tissues as well as archival cytologic smears or paraffin-embedded tissue sections. This also allows FISH to be utilized in the differentiation of signals from cells in healthy and cancerous conditions as well as in the enhancement of "interphase cytogenetics" in both tumor and prenatal settings.

FISH is often used in interpretation of numerical and complex chromosome aberrations and the evaluation of HER2/neu oncogene amplification in breast carcinoma and for detection of different translocations in chronic myelogenous leukemia and acute myelogenous leukemia.

Spectral Karyotyping Imaging

Spectral karyotyping imaging (SKI) is a cytogenetic technique, developed by Schrock et al. (1996) and it combined the two basic principles of FISH which are chromosome painting and multicolor fluorescence. This involves the use of 24 sets of chromosome-specific "painting" probes. SKI is based on the labeling of each probe with varying proportions of five fluorochromes, differently combined for each specific chromosome in a light of unique spectral emission. This enables the display and identification of all 24 human chromosomes assigned in different colors in a single metaphase, by using a combination of probe labeling, fluorescence microscopy, spectroscopy, CCD-imaging and spectral image analysis without prior knowledge of abnormalities involved.

This technology allows the use of an "interferometer" like those used by astronomers for differentiating light spectra emitted by different stars. The slight variations in color, undetectable by the human eye, are detected by this computerized device. This then reassigns an easy-to-distinguish visual color (classification color) to each pair of chromosomes.

Despite the analytical importance of SKI, the following limitations have been reported:

❖ Structural abnormalities, such as inversion, deletion, insertion, and duplication in the same chromosome are shown with the same color thus, impossible to evaluate.

- Also, the Q-positive segment and the satellite region of the long arm of the Y chromosome near the centromere cannot be detected.

Moreover, the development of spectral color banding technique has overcome the limitations of SKI and this technique combine G-band differential staining with the SKI coloring technology. The widespread clinical use of SKI in the field of clinical genetics has made significant contributions in molecular diagnosis of disorders but the cost of this technique remains a drawback.

DNA Microarrays

Microarray refers to a small, two-dimensional high-density matrix of DNA fragments which are printed or synthesized on a glass or silicon slide (chip) in a specific order. Deoxyribonucleic acid (DNA) microarrays **(Fig. 2.5)** can be utilized for gene expression and simultaneous assessment of the expression rate of multiple genes in a particular sample. The two types of DNA microarrays that are widely used are cDNA microarrays and oligonucleotide/DNA chips. In cDNA microarrays, DNA sequences complementary to arrays of mRNA from multiple genes are mechanically placed on a single glass slide. This is followed by specific attachment of the immobilized cDNA sequences serving as anchoring probes to which mRNA are extracted from the tested sample during hybridization. The tagging of the tested mRNA with a fluorescent dye produces fluorescence at each anchoring probe location, the intensity of which is proportional to the amount of mRNA (expression degree) of the gene at that location.

A microarray reader normally displays the intensity of fluorescence at each cDNA location as a colored dot per gene location on a grid. This computerized reader is linked to a database that indicates the gene at each intercept location.

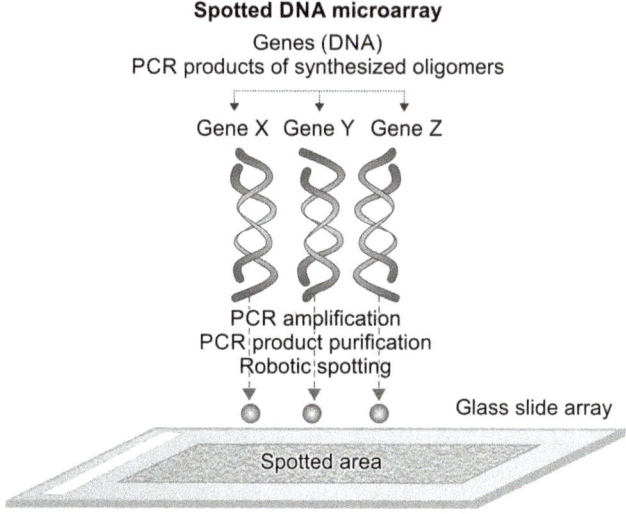

Fig. 2.5: DNA microarray.

Oligonucleotide/DNA chips comprise silicon chips on which the "anchoring" oligonucleotide sequences are directly synthesized. This silicon chips serve as the immobilized probes to which the complementary specific mRNA will hybridize. DNA chips can be produced with large density of gene arrays encoding up to 12,000 or more genes on a single chip.

The DNA microarrays technique has been utilized in the analysis and comparison of numerous tumor samples through the building of gene expression "fingerprints" databases and linking of specific patterns of expression to primary site of origin, prognosis and outcome of therapy.

POLYMERASE CHAIN REACTION

Polymerase chain reaction (PCR) is a revolutionary method developed in 1983 by Kary Mullis. PCR has proved to be a valuable method and remained the most frequently used molecular technique in molecular pathology laboratories and it is an extremely versatile technique for copying DNA with the aid of DNA polymerase.

In this technique, the predetermined copying or modification of a specific DNA sequence and identification of DNA fragment in a cDNA library is enhanced by DNA polymerase enzyme, which amplifies the specific fragments of the target DNA molecule added to the reaction. These nucleotides are named as primers and contain the sequences complementary to the target sequences of the target DNA molecule. The PCR technique can also be used to introduce restriction enzyme sites to ends of DNA molecules, or to change bases of DNA (referred to as site-directed mutagenesis)

The sequence of reactions in PCR is extremely powerful such that amplification of a DNA molecule produces about 1 billion molecules under a short period of time (<2 hours) as the reaction is done under perfect conditions.

PCR has different role such as reverse transcription PCR (RT-PCR) for amplification of RNA and quantitative PCR which allow for quantitative measurement of DNA or RNA molecules. Multiple copies of a targeted chimeric gene can be obtained by using a pair of priming complementary sequences (oligonucleotide primers) together with unique heat-resistant polymerases (DNA copying enzymes).

The Multiplex PCR (mPCR) which is employed for the simultaneous identification of several gene sequences belonging to the same pathogen or originating from a mixture of different pathogens.

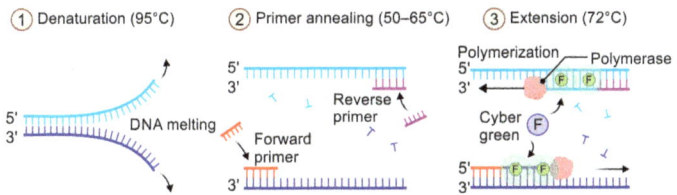

Fig. 2.6: Polymerase chain reaction (PCR).

Each PCR cycle involves three basic steps: **Denaturing, annealing (or hybridization), and Extension (polymerization) (Fig. 2.6).**

During denaturing, the 2 strands of the helix of the target genetic (DNA) material are unwound and separated by heating at 90° to 95°C. During annealing, there is binding of oligonucleotide primers to their complementary bases on the single-stranded DNA. This step requires a much cooler temperature, 55°C. Finally, during extension (at 72°C), the template strand is read by polymerase and is paired rapidly with the appropriate nucleotides, resulting in 2 new helices consisting of part of the original strand and the complementary strand that was just assembled. The process is repeated 30 to 40 times, with doubling of the amount of the targeted genetic material in each cycle. At the end of the procedure, multiple identical copies (in millions) of the original specific DNA sequence would be produced. The copies are expected to migrate concurrently when subjected to electrophoresis to form a single band due to their similarities in electrical charge and molecular weight.

The specificity of a PCR assay is determined by the target DNA sequence under evaluation, the sequence of the oligonucleotide probe, similar sequences that may exist elsewhere in nature and the intentions of the assay designer.

REAL TIME PCR AND RT PCR

In real-time PCR, the amount of DNA is measured after each cycle via fluorescent dyes that yield increasing fluorescent signal in direct proportion to the number of PCR product molecules (amplicons) generated. Data collected in the exponential phase of the reaction yield quantitative information on the starting quantity of the amplification target. Fluorescent reporters used in real time PCR include double-stranded DNA (dsDNA)- binding dyes, or dye molecules attached to PCR primers or probes that hybridize with PCR product during amplification. The change in fluorescence over the course of the reaction is measured by an instrument that combines thermal cycling with fluorescent dye scanning capability. By plotting fluorescence against the cycle number, the real-time PCR instrument generates an amplification plot that represents the accumulation of product over the duration of the entire PCR reaction.

The Advantages of Real-time PCR Include

- Ability to monitor the progress of the PCR reaction as it occurs in real time.
- Ability to precisely measure the amount of amplicon at each cycle, which allows highly accurate quantification of the amount of starting material in samples.
- An increased dynamic range of detection.
- Amplification and detection occur in a single tube, eliminating post-PCR manipulations. Over the past several years, real-time PCR has become the leading tool for the detection and quantification of DNA or RNA. Using these techniques, you can achieve precise detection that is accurate within a two-fold range, with a dynamic range of input material covering 6 to 8 orders of magnitude.

Two-step qRT-PCR

Two-step quantitative reverse transcriptase PCR (qRT-PCR) starts with the reverse transcription of either total RNA or poly(A)+ RNA into cDNA using a reverse transcriptase (RT). This first-strand cDNA synthesis reaction can be primed using random primers, oligo (dT), or gene-specific primers (GSPs). The temperature used for cDNA synthesis depends on the RT enzyme chosen. Next, approximately 10% of the cDNA is transferred to a separate tube for the real-time PCR reaction.

One-step qRT-PCR

One-step qRT-PCR combines the first-strand cDNA synthesis reaction and real-time PCR reaction in the same tube, simplifying reaction setup and reducing the possibility of contamination. Gene-specific primers (GSP) are required. This is because using oligo(dT) or random primers will generate nonspecific products in the one-step procedure and reduce the amount of product of interest.

PCR COMPONENTS

DNA Polymerase

DNA polymerases are a group of enzymes required for DNA synthesis. Arthur Kornberg purified and characterized DNA polymerase from *E.coli* for the first time. It is a single-chain polypeptide now known as DNA polymerase-I **(Fig. 2.7)**.

The main function of the DNA polymerase is to synthesize DNA by the process of replication. It is an important process to maintain and transfer genetic information from one generation to another. DNA polymerase works in pairs, replicating two strands of DNA in

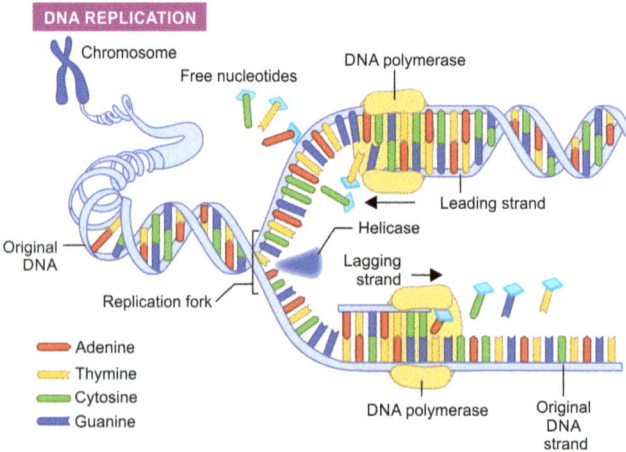

Fig. 2.7: DNA polymerase.

tandem. They add deoxyribonucleotides at the 3'–OH group of the growing DNA strand. The DNA strand grows in 5' → 3' direction by their polymerization activity. Adenine pairs with thymine and guanine pairs with cytosine. DNA polymerases cannot initiate the replication process and they need a primer to add to the nucleotides.

Reverse Transcriptase

A reverse transcriptase (RT) is an enzyme that is used in the process of reverse transcription and is used to synthesize DNA (circular DNA or cDNA) from RNA. This enzyme reverse transcriptase is available in certain infections that have the hereditary material as the RNA. It is needed for the reverse record of the viral RNA to

DNA further which can be embedded into the host DNA. Hence, the enzyme in RNA-dependent DNA polymerase, in which the RNA section is considered as the parent and the cDNA is incorporated.

The reverse transcriptase (RT) is as critical to the success of qRT-PCR as the DNA polymerase. It is important to choose an RT that not only provides high yields of full-length cDNA, but also has good activity at high temperatures. High-temperature performance is also very important for denaturation of RNA with secondary structure. In one-step qRT-PCR, an RT that retains its activity at higher temperatures allows to use a PCR with a high melting temperature (Tm), increasing specificity and reducing background.

DNTPs

Nucleotides are basic building blocks of nucleic acids. It consists of a sugar molecule (DNA or RNA), a nitrogenous base and a phosphate group. The nitrogenous bases are adenine (A), guanine (G), cytosine (C), thymine (T) and uracil (U). dNTP or deoxyribonucleotides contain deoxyribose as the sugar molecule. The nitrogenous bases are either purines or pyrimidines that interact through hydrogen bonds to form base pairs and carry genetic information. The four dNTPs are dATP, dCTP, dGTP and dTTP. dNTP is a building block of a PCR Chain. Each DNTP contain dNTP of each ATGC sequence.

Magnesium Concentration

$MgCl_2$ (Magnesium chloride) is an essential ingredient of the PCR master mix. Acting as a cofactor, it enhances the enzymatic activity of DNA polymerase, thereby boosting DNA amplification. $MgCl_2$ has functions in both facilitating Taq DNA polymerase activity and primer annealing specificity on the template DNA/RNA strand.

Primers

It is set of oligonucleotide initiate the PCR reaction. In the PCR method, a pair of primers hybridizes with the sample DNA and defines the region that will be amplified, resulting in millions and millions of copies in a very short timeframe.

Probes

A probe is pieces of DNA (oligonucleotides) complimentary to the template and labeled with a fluorescent dye.

TaqMan Probe

TaqMan probes are oligonucleotides that have a fluorescent probe attached to the 5' end and a quencher to the 3' end. During PCR amplification, these probes will hybridize to the target sequences located in the amplicon and as polymerase replicates the template with TaqMan bound, it also cleaves the fluorescent probe due to polymerase 5'-nuclease activity. Because the proximity between the quench molecule and the fluorescent probe normally prevents fluorescence from being detected through FRET, the decoupling results in the increase of intensity of fluorescence proportional to the number of the probe cleavage cycles. Although well-designed TaqMan probes produce accurate real-time RT-PCR results.

Template

The sample DNA that contains the target sequence. At the beginning of the reaction, high temperature is applied to the original double-stranded DNA molecule to separate the strands from each other.

RNAse/Nuclease Free Water

Nuclease-free water is free of both DNAse and RNAse, and involves treating with DEPC (diethylpyrocarbonate) and/or autoclaving to inactivate RNAse and DNAse. Ultrapure water, on the other hand, is obtained by ultrafiltration to achieve the high level of purity. It also does not contain any nucleases.

Master Mix

A PCR master mix, sometimes known as super mix or ready mix, is a batch mixture of PCR reagents at optimal concentrations that can be prepared and divided among many PCR tubes or 96-well PCR plates. The master mix usually includes DNA polymerase, dNTPs, $MgCl_2$ and buffer. Using a master mix reduces pipetting and risk of contamination, is convenient, saves time and pre-empts possible errors in mixing, making it ideal for high-throughput applications. The master mix enables researchers to set up controls and test different concentrations of their target DNA or RNA templates without having to individually add precise amounts of enzymes, buffers, cofactor (usually $MgCl_2$), water and dNTP to each reaction tube or plate well. Instead, a large master mix containing all or most of the PCR reagents is prepared once. The appropriate amount of master mix can be pipetted into tubes or plate wells and combined with any components that vary among the reactions, such as DNA or RNA templates or primers.

Cycle Threshold (Ct)

In a real time PCR assay a positive reaction is detected by accumulation of a fluorescent signal. The cycle threshold (Ct) is defined as the number of cycles required for the fluorescent signal to cross the threshold (i.e., exceeds background level). Ct levels are inversely proportional to the amount of target nucleic acid in the sample (i.e., the lower the Ct level the greater the amount of target nucleic acid in the sample).

Nucleic Acid Extraction

Nucleic acid extraction is the first step of any amplification experiment no matter what kind of amplification is used to detect a specific pathogen. It is a crucial preanalytic step in the development and performance of any successful molecular diagnostic method and ensures a reliable result. Nucleic acid extraction consists of three major processes: isolation, purification, and concentration. Ideally, the final target is pure nucleic acid without amplification inhibitors or contaminants such as protein, carbohydrate, and other nucleic acids.

Nucleic Acid Extraction Techniques

Cesium Chloride/Ethidium Bromide Density Gradient Centrifugation

Since 1950, density gradient centrifugation using cesium chloride (CsCl)/ethidium bromide (EtBr) has been used as for DNA extraction method and has become standard in research laboratories. The basic principle of this method is to use the difference in density between the cesium ion and water and intercalation of EtBr, which shows good results for separation of various DNAs and the procurement of high-yield DNA. For example, each DNA can be separated as independent bands as a result of the differences in each DNA's density in the gradient by the intercalation of EtBr. However, it has important limitations in that it requires an expensive ultracentrifuge and considerable time, it is difficult to perform, and EtBr is harmful. Consequently, this method is not suitable for clinical microbiology and has not been used in the clinical laboratory.

Phenol–Chloroform Extraction

Phenol–chloroform extraction is widely used. The process consists of vigorous mixing of phenol–chloroform solution and sample followed by centrifugation. Phenol does not completely inhibit RNase activity, and this characteristic enables isolation of nucleic acid by combination with chloroform and alcohol. After centrifugation, the upper (aqueous) phase containing the DNA can be separated from the lower (organic) phase containing denatured proteins, and DNA can be precipitated by adding ethanol or isopropanol with a high concentration of salt. After washing with 70% ethanol to remove any remaining ethanol or isopropanol, the final target DNA is collected by dissolving it in TE buffer or sterile distilled water. This method is also used for RNA extraction by concomitant use of guanidinium isothiocyanate. This combination can overcome the limitation of RNA extraction using the guanidinium isothiocyanate itself, so RNA could be isolated conveniently using a single-step technique by Chomczynski et al. Total RNA is recovered by precipitation with isopropanol after separation of the upper phase containing the total RNA from the lower phase containing DNA and proteins. Although the phenol–chloroform method is relatively easy compared with CsCl/EtBr and is very useful for the extraction of nucleic acids, it is problematic for the clinical microbiology laboratory because phenol has important limitations due to it being toxic, caustic, and flammable.

Solid-Phase Extraction (Spin Column Method) (Fig. 2.8)

Solid-phase extraction uses a spin column operated by centrifugal force allowing DNA to be purified rapidly and efficiently without the limitations of liquid extraction, including incomplete phase separation. Solid-phase extraction using silica now is one of the most common methods for nucleic acid extraction. Silica that possesses a positive charge combines strongly with DNA, which possesses a negative charge, so it can enable rapid, pure, and quantitative purification. In 1990, Boom et al. used an innovative approach

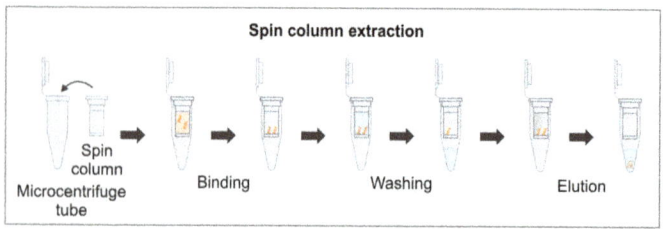

Fig. 2.8: Spin column method.

in which diatomaceous earth served as a matrix for solid-phase extraction. The principle of this method is that it immobilizes DNA onto its particles in the presence of a chaotropic agent. The technique can purify rRNA as well as single-stranded and double-stranded DNA. It takes only a short time and can be applied to clinical specimens as well as to DNA and bacteria. The process of solid-phase extraction involves cell lysis, nucleic acid adsorption, washing, and elution. Column conditioning is obtained using a buffer at a particular pH. The nucleic acid will be released after cell lysis and decanting of lysis buffer into the column. Nucleic acid adsorption is completed in a chaotropic salt solution. Washing buffer contains a competitive agent and can remove contaminants such as proteins and salts. In elution, TE buffer is applied to the column so that purified nucleic acid will be released.

Magnetic Bead Method (Fig. 2.9)

There is another important modification of solid-phase extraction, that is, the magnetic bead method. The beads have a negative surface charge and bind proteins and cellular debris selectively. So, DNA can be isolated easily from specimens by removing proteins and cellular debris on the beads. This has the potential advantages of removing

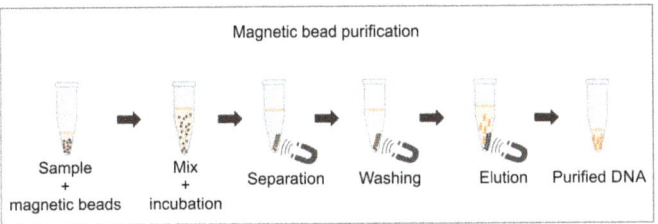

Fig. 2.9: Magnetic bead method.

the need for repeated centrifugation, vacuum filtration, and column separation for washing and elution as well as organic solvents. The magnetic bead method is very simple and convenient; so many commercial kits are available for this method. Some manufacturers combined the techniques of solid-phase extraction using silica and magnetic beads, which satisfies the customers requests for time- and labor-effectiveness and efficiency. This method is commonly used in automated extraction methods such as miniMag (bioMerieux) and MagNA Pure (Roche). In terms of new technology, additional commercial kits using this new technique are being launched into the market. The enzymatic method is an example of these new extraction methods. These new methods help investigators by giving advantages of more convenience, requirement for only small volumes of specimen, and enhancement of DNA recovery.

REAL-TIME PCR ANALYSIS AND TROUBLESHOOTING

This section defines the major terms used in real-time PCR analysis.

Baseline

The baseline of the real-time PCR reaction refers to the signal level during the initial cycles of PCR, usually cycles **(Fig. 2.10)**

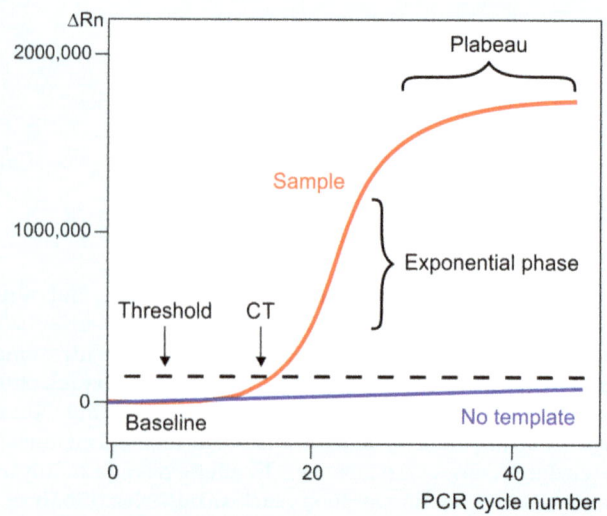

Fig. 2.10: PCR cycle.

3 to 15, in which there is little change in fluorescent signal. The low-level signal of the baseline can be equated to the background or the "noise" of the reaction. The baseline in real-time PCR is determined empirically for each reaction, by user analysis or automated analysis of the amplification plot. The baseline should be set carefully to allow accurate determination of the threshold cycle (Ct), defined below. The baseline determination should take into account enough cycles to eliminate the background found in

the early cycles of amplification but should not include the cycles in which the amplification signal begins to rise above background. When comparing different real time PCR reactions or experiments, the baseline should be defined in the same way for each.

Threshold

The threshold of the real-time PCR reaction is the level of signal that reflects a statistically significant increase over the calculated baseline signal. It is set to distinguish relevant amplification signal from the background. Usually, real-time PCR instrument software automatically sets the threshold at 10 times the standard deviation of the fluorescence value of the baseline. However, the positioning of the threshold can be set at any point in the exponential phase of PCR.

Threshold Cycle

The threshold cycle (Ct) **(Fig. 2.11)** is the cycle number at which the fluorescent signal of the reaction crosses the threshold. The Ct is used to calculate the initial DNA copy number, because the Ct value is inversely related to the starting amount of target. For example, in comparing real-time PCR results from samples containing different amounts of target, a sample with twice the starting amount will yield a Ct one cycle earlier than a sample that contained half as many copies of the target prior to amplification. This assumes that the PCR is operating at 100% efficiency (i.e., the amount of product doubles perfectly during each cycle) in both reactions. As the template amount decreases, the cycle number at which significant amplification is seen increases.

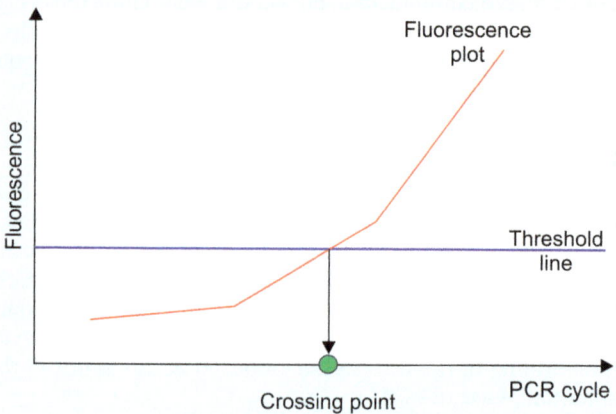

Fig. 2.11: The threshold cycle (Ct).

Standard Curve (Fig. 2.12)

A dilution series of known template concentrations can be used to establish a standard curve for determining the initial starting amount of the target template in experimental samples or for assessing the reaction efficiency. The log of each known concentration in the dilution series (X-axis) is plotted against the Ct value for that concentration (Y-axis). From this standard curve, information about the performance of the reaction as well as various reaction parameters (including slope, y-intercept, and correlation coefficient) can be derived. The concentrations chosen for the standard curve should encompass the expected concentration range of the target in the experimental samples.

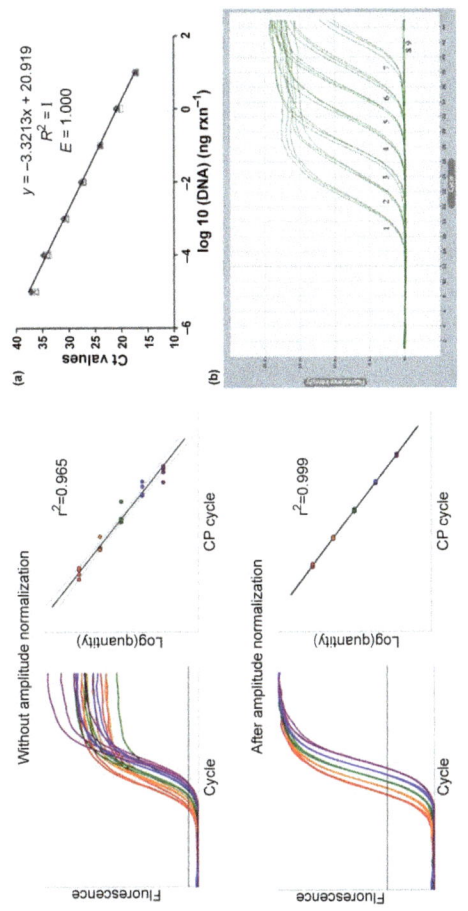

Fig. 2.12: Standard curve.

Correlation coefficient (R^2) (Fig. 2.13)

The correlation coefficient is a measure of how well the data fit the standard curve. The R^2 value reflects the linearity of the standard curve. Ideally, $R^2 = 1$, although 0.999 is generally the maximum value.

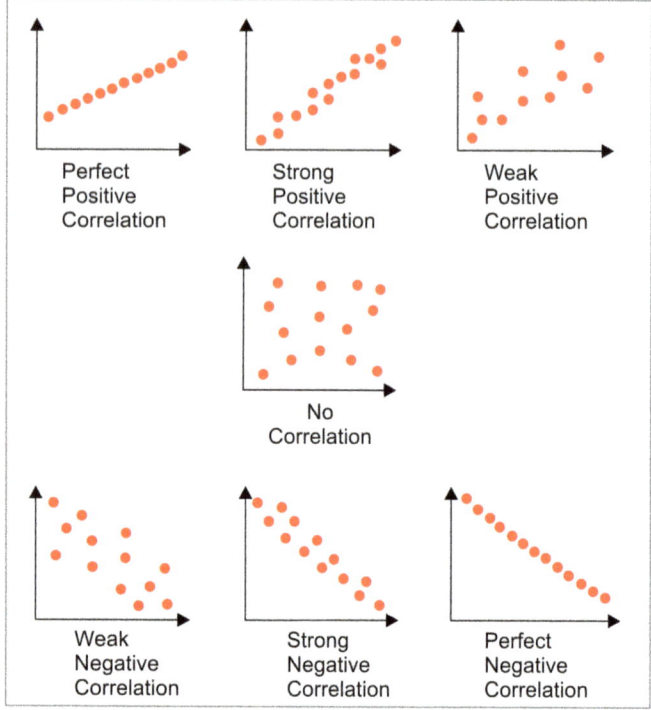

Fig. 2.13: Correlation coefficient (R^2).

Y-intercept (Fig. 2.14)

The y-intercept corresponds to the theoretical limit of detection of the reaction, or the CT value expected if the lowest copy number of target molecules denoted on the X-axis gave rise to statistically significant amplification. Though PCR is theoretically capable of detecting a single copy of a target, a copy number of 2–10 is commonly specified as the lowest target level that can be reliably quantified in real-time PCR applications. This limits the usefulness of the y-intercept value as a direct measure of sensitivity. However, the y-intercept value may be useful for comparing different amplification systems and targets.

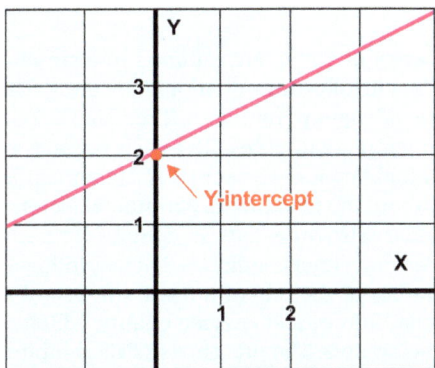

Fig. 2.14: Y-intercept.

Exponential Phase

It is important to quantify your real-time PCR reaction in the early part of the exponential phase as opposed to in the later cycles or when the reaction reaches the plateau. At the beginning of the exponential phase, all reagents are still in excess, the DNA polymerase is still highly efficient, and the amplification product, which is present in a low amount, will not compete with the primers' annealing capabilities. All of these things contribute to more accurate data.

Slope

The slope of the log-linear phase of the amplification reaction is a measure of reaction efficiency. To obtain accurate and reproducible results, reactions should have an efficiency as close to 100% as possible, equivalent to a slope of –3.32 (see **Fig. 2.15**, for more detail).

Efficiency

A PCR efficiency of 100% corresponds to a slope of –3.32, as determined by the following equation: Efficiency = 10 (–1/slope) –1 ideally, the efficiency (E) of a PCR reaction should be 100%, meaning the template doubles after each thermal cycle during exponential amplification. The actual efficiency can give valuable information about the reaction. Experimental factors such as the length, secondary structure, and GC content of the amplicon can influence efficiency. Other conditions that may influence efficiency are the dynamics of the reaction itself, the use of nonoptimal reagent concentrations, and enzyme quality, which can result in efficiencies below 90%. The presence of PCR inhibitors in one or more of the reagents can produce efficiencies of greater than 110%. A good reaction should have an efficiency between 90% and 110%, which corresponds to a slope of between –3.58 and –3.10.

Dynamic Range

This is the range over which an increase in starting material concentration results in a corresponding increase in amplification

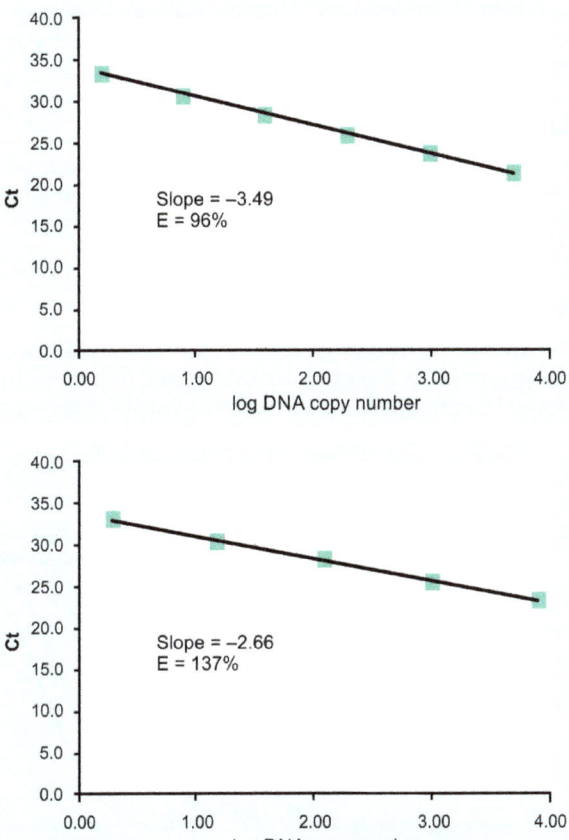

Fig. 2.15: Slope of the log-linear phase.

product. Ideally, the dynamic range for real-time PCR should be 7–8 orders of magnitude for plasmid DNA and at least a 3–4 log range for cDNA or genomic DNA.

Absolute Quantification

Absolute quantification describes a real-time PCR experiment in which samples of known quantity are serially diluted and then amplified to generate a standard curve. Unknown samples are then quantified by comparison with this curve.

Relative Quantification

Relative quantification (**Fig. 2.16**) describes a real-time PCR experiment in which the expression of a gene of interest in one sample (i.e., treated) is compared to expression of the same gene in another sample (i.e., untreated). The results are expressed as fold change (increase or decrease) in expression of the treated in relation

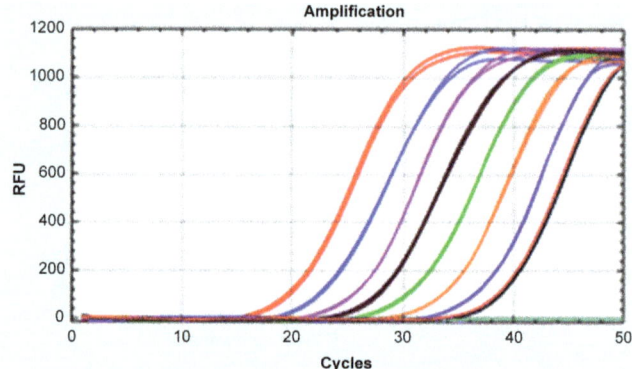

Fig. 2.16: Relative quantification.

to the untreated. A normalizer gene (such as β-actin) is used as a control for experimental variability in this type of quantification.

Melting Curve (Dissociation Curve)

A melting curve charts the change in fluorescence observed when double-stranded DNA (dsDNA) with incorporated dye molecules dissociate, or "melts" into single-stranded DNA (ssDNA) as the temperature of the reaction is raised. For example, when double-stranded DNA bound with SYBR®Green I dye is heated, a sudden decrease in fluorescence is detected when the melting point (Tm) is reached, due to dissociation of the DNA strands and subsequent release of the dye. The fluorescence is plotted against temperature.

Real-time PCR Fluorescence Detection Systems (Fig. 2.17)

Many real-time fluorescent PCR chemistries exist, but the most widely used are the 5 nuclease assay; the most well-known of which is the TaqMan® Assay and SYBR® Green dye-based assays.

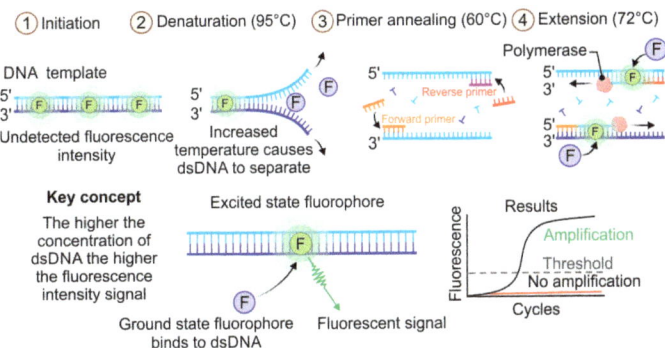

Fig. 2.17: Fluorescent dye-based real-time PCR.

The 5' nuclease domain can degrade DNA bound to the template, downstream of DNA synthesis. A second key element in the 5' nuclease assay is a phenomenon called FRET: fluorescent resonance energy transfer. In FRET, the emissions of a fluorescent dye can be strongly reduced by the presence of another dye, often called the quencher, in proximity.

Taqman® Probe Types

5' nuclease assay offer two tools for specificity: primers and probes. For maximal impact on specificity by primers, a mismatch between the target and homolog must be positioned at the 3'-most base of the primer. A mismatch further away from the 3' end may have little to no impact on specificity. In contrast, mismatches across most of the length of a MGB probe, which is shorter than a TaqMan® probe (**Fig. 2.18**), can have a strong impact on specificity—TaqMan® MGB probes are stronger tools for specificity than primers.

Reference Dye

Most real-time PCR reactions contain multiple dyes, e.g., one or more reporter dyes, in some cases a quencher dye, and, very often, a passive reference dye. Multiple dyes in the same well can be measured independently, either through optimized combinations of excitation and emission filters or through a process called multicomponenting. Multicomponenting is a mathematical method to measure dye intensity for each dye in the reaction. Multicomponenting offers the benefits of easy correction for dye designation errors, refreshing optical performance to factory standard without hardware adjustment, and provides a source of troubleshooting information. The basic dye available is FAM, CY5, HEX, VIC, Texas Red, Alexa, ATTO.

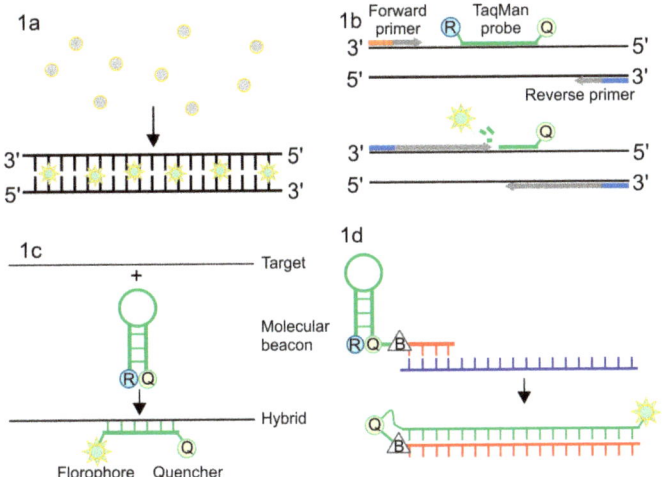

Fig. 2.18: TaqMan® probes.

Reference Control and Reference Gene

Controls in real-time PCR reactions prove that signal obtained from experimental samples represent the amplicon of interest, thereby validating specificity. All experiments should include a no-template control (NTC), and qRT-PCR reactions should also include a no-reverse transcriptase control (no-RT).

NTC controls should contain all reaction components except the DNA or cDNA sample. Amplification detected in these wells is due to either primer-dimers or contamination with completed PCR reaction product. This type of contamination can make expression levels look higher than they actually are. No-RT reactions should contain all reaction components except the reverse transcriptase. If amplification products are seen in no-RT control reactions, it indicates that DNA was amplified rather than cDNA. This can also artificially inflate apparent expression levels in experimental samples.

The use of a normalizer gene (also called a reference gene or endogenous control) is the most thorough method of addressing almost every source of variability in real-time PCR. However, for this method to work, the gene must be present at a consistent level in all samples being compared. An effective normalizer gene controls for RNA quality and quantity, and differences in both RT and real-time PCR amplification efficiencies. If the RT transcribes or the DNA polymerase amplifies a target at different rates in two different samples, the normalizer transcript will reflect that variability. Endogenous reference genes, such as a "housekeeping" gene, or exogenous nucleic acid targets can be used.

Endogenous Controls Common endogenous normalizers in real-time PCR include:

- **β-actin (BACT):** Cytoskeletal gene
- **18S ribosomal RNA (rRNA):** Ribosomal subunit
- **Cyclophilin A (CYC):** Serine-threonine phosphatase inhibitor
- **Glyceraldehyde phosphate dehydrogenase (GAPDH):** Glycolysis pathway

GAPDH is a common normalizer that has been shown to be consistent in many cases. However, GAPDH is upregulated in some cancerous cells, in cells treated with tumor suppressors, under hypoxic conditions, and in manganese or insulin-treated samples.

Exogenous normalizers: Exogenous normalizers are not as commonly employed but are a viable alternative if a highly consistent endogenous normalizer cannot be found for a specific sample set. An exogenous reference gene is a synthetic or in vitro transcribed

RNA whose sequence is not present in the experimental samples. Due to its exogenous origin, it does not undergo the normal biological fluctuations that can occur in a cell under different conditions or treatments.

The drawbacks to employing an exogenous normalizer are.
- It's not endogenous. Maximize the utility of exogenous normalizers by spiking them into the workflow early, for example into the cell lysis buffer.
- Accuracy is subject to pipetting variability when introducing the normalizer.
- Transcript stability may be affected by prolonged storage and multiple freeze-thaws. Therefore, copy number should be routinely assessed to ensure it has not shifted over time.

Multiplex Real-time PCR (Fig. 2.19)

PCR multiplexing is the amplification and specific detection of two or more genetic sequences in the same reaction. To be successful, PCR multiplexing must be able to produce sufficient amplified product for the detection of all the intended sequences using an endpoint detection method, such as gel electrophoresis. PCR multiplexing is used for qualitative results. Real-time PCR multiplexing may be used to produce qualitative or quantitative results. To be successful for real-time quantitative PCR multiplexing, sufficient geometric phase signal for all the intended sequences must be produced. The suffix "plex" is used in multiple terms. Singleplex is an assay designed to amplify a single genetic sequence. Duplex is an assay designed to amplify two genetic sequences. The most common type of multiplex is a duplex, in which the assay for the target gene is conducted in the same well as that for the control or normalizer gene.

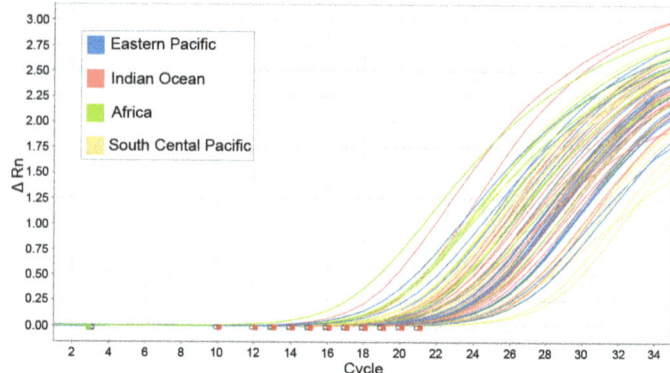

Fig. 2.19: Multiplex real-time PCR.

Multiplexing Benefits

Three benefits of multiplexing, increased throughput (more samples potentially assayed per plate), reduced sample usage, and reduced reagent usage, are dependent on the number of targets in the experiment.

For example, if a quantitative experiment consists of only one target assay, running the target assay as a duplex with the normalizer assay will increase throughput, reduce sample, and reduce reagent usage by 2-fold. However, if a quantitative experiment consists of two target assays, two duplexes would be needed to produce all the data.

Instrumentation for Multiplexing

Multiplex assays usually involve multiple dyes in the same well. The real-time PCR instrument must be capable of measuring those different dye signals in the same well with accuracy. These measurements must remain specific for each dye, even when one dye signal is significantly higher than another.

Chemistry Recommendations for Multiplexing

The best fluorescent chemistries for real-time PCR multiplexing are those that can assign different dyes to detect each genetic sequence in the multiplex. Most of the multiplexing is performed with multi-dye, high specificity chemistries, such as TaqMan® probe-based assays.

Dye Choices for Multiplexing

Assuming a multi-dye real-time PCR fluorescent chemistry is being used, each genetic sequence being detected in the multiplex will require a different reporter dye. The reporter dyes chosen must be sufficiently excited and accurately detected when together in the same well by the real-time PCR instrument. The instrument manufacturer should be able to offer dye recommendations.

Chapter 2: PCRs-Technology, Techniques, History and Challenges

LIST OF TROUBLESHOOTING GRAPHS

1. Valid Graph (Fig. 2.20)

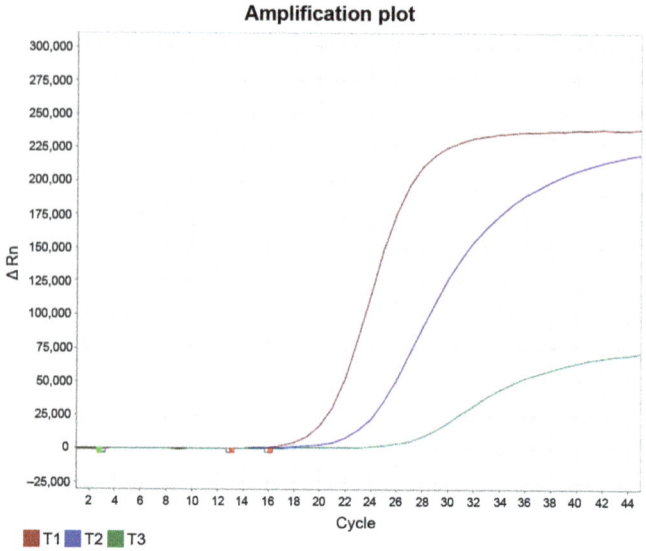

Fig. 2.20: Valid graph.

2. Invalid Graph (Fig. 2.21)

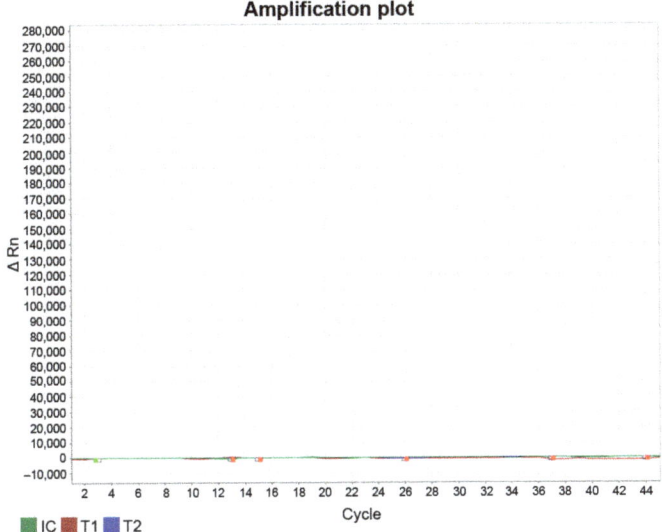

Fig. 2.21: Invalid graph.

Possible Causes

- Incorrectly assigned reporter dye.
- Pipetting errors and improper handling of reagents.
- Error during sample extraction.
- Presence of inhibitors.
- Degraded reagents.

Solutions

- Check the protocol and details mentioned on the package insert.
- Repeat the test. Ensure that the pipettes are calibrated.
- Check quality of the sample and extraction protocol. Re-extract the sample if required.
- Ensure there are no inhibitors in the extracted sample.
- Check the quality/stability of reagents and Instrument by testing with positive controls.

3. Valid without Amplification in IC (Fig. 2.22)

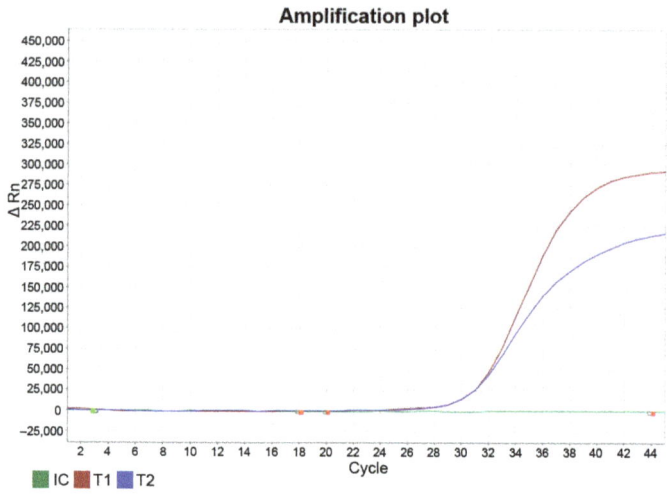

Fig. 2.22: Valid without amplification in IC.

Possible Causes
- ❖ Pipetting errors and improper handling of reagents.
- ❖ Very old sample used for testing.
- ❖ Presence of inhibitors.

Solutions
- ❖ Repeat the test. Ensure that the pipettes are calibrated.
- ❖ Check quality of the sample and extraction protocol. Re-extract the sample if required.
- ❖ Ensure there are no inhibitors in the sample.
- ❖ Ensure that all required dye are working in the instrument.

4. Low Amplitude and High Amplitude (Figs. 2.23 and 2.24)

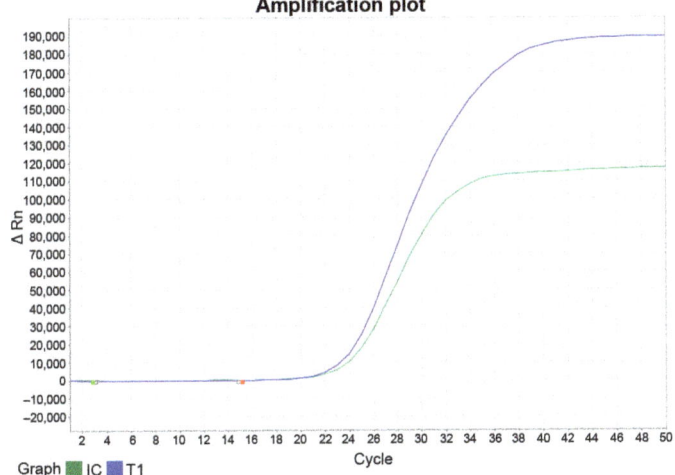

Fig. 2.23: Low amplitude.

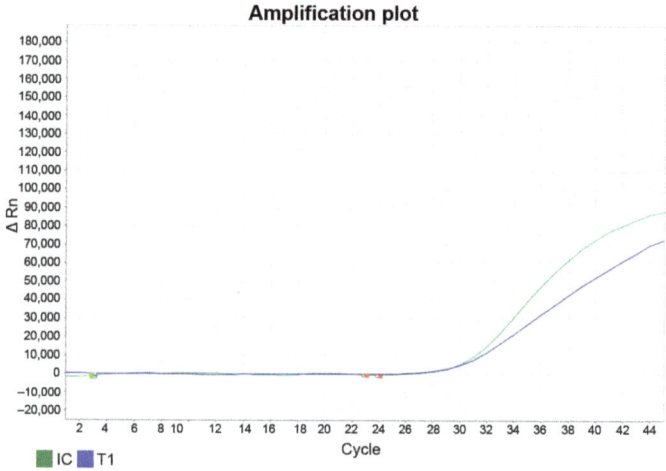

Fig. 2.24: High amplitude.

Possible Causes

- Pipetting errors and improper handling of reagents.
- Presence of inhibitors.

Solutions

- Repeat the test. Ensure that the pipettes are calibrated.
- Check quality of the sample and extraction protocol. Re-extract the sample if required.
- Ensure there are no inhibitors in the sample.
- Check the amplitude of curve with respected dye positive control.

5. High Background Noise Graph (Fig. 2.25)

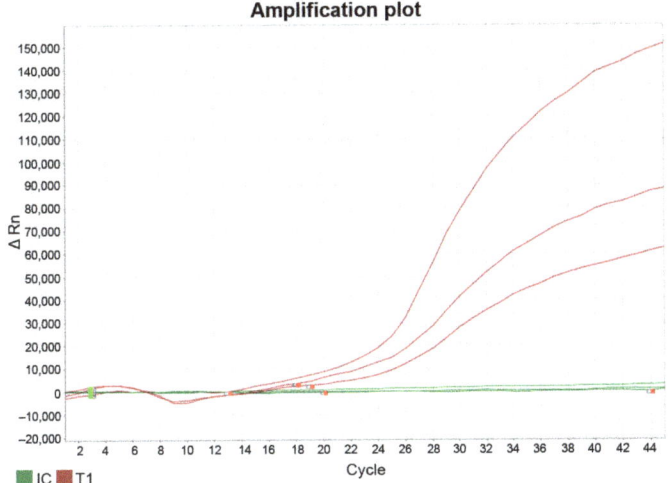

Fig. 2.25: High background noise graph.

Possible Causes
- Presence of inhibitors.
- Presence of degraded probe.
- Inappropriate auto-scaling and baseline settings by the instrument software.
- Too much template added to the reaction.

Solutions
- Check the quality of the sample and ensure there are no inhibitors in the sample.

- Check the quality/stability of reagents by testing with positive controls.
- Adjust the baseline settings according to appropriate cycles on the instrument software.
- Repeat the test with fresh sample. Dilute the sample if required.

6. Graph Dropping below Zero then Showing Amplification (Fig. 2.26)

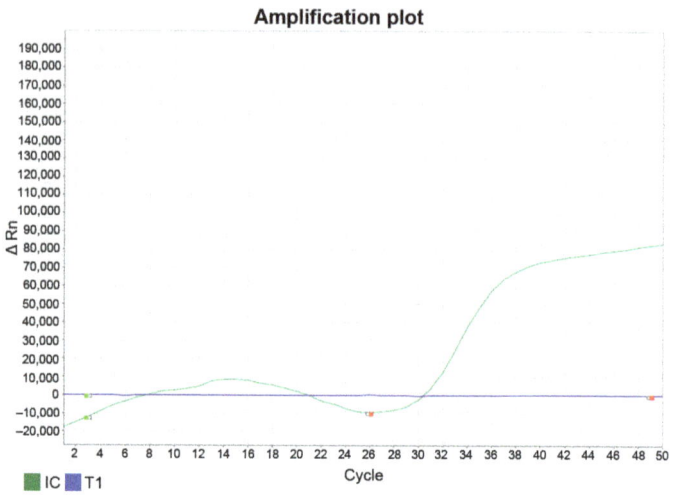

Fig. 2.26: Graph dropping below zero then showing amplification.

Possible Causes
- Presence of inhibitors.
- Presence of degraded probe.

- Inappropriate auto-scaling and baseline settings by the instrument software.

Solutions
- Check sample quality and ensure there are no inhibitors in the sample.
- Check the quality/stability of reagents by testing with positive controls.
- Adjust the baseline settings according to appropriate cycles on the instrument software.

7. Distorted Graph (Fig. 2.27)

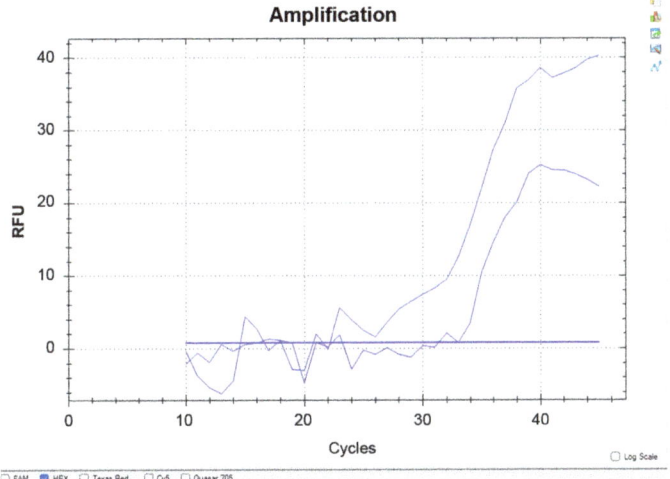

Fig. 2.27: Distorted graph.

Possible Causes

- Incorrectly assigned reporter dye.
- Passive reference not set as "None".
- Pipetting errors and improper handling of reagents.
- Very old sample used for testing.
- Presence of inhibitors.
- Inappropriate auto-scaling and baseline settings by the instrument software.

Solutions

- Check the protocol and details mentioned in the package insert.
- Set the passive reference as "None" and re-analyze the data in the software.
- Repeat the test. Ensure that the pipettes are calibrated.
- Check the extraction protocol and re-extract the sample if required.
- Check sample quality and ensure there are no inhibitors in the sample.
- Adjust the baseline settings according to appropriate cycles on the instrument software.

8. Ideal Calibrator Graph (Fig. 2.28)

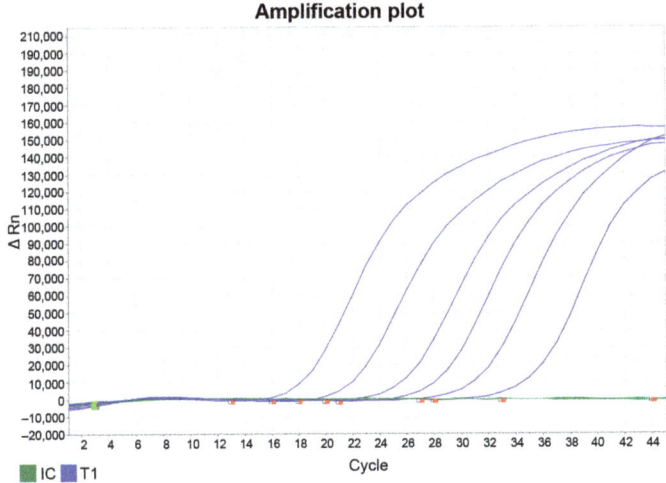

Fig. 2.28: Ideal calibrator graph.

9. Inconsistent Spacing in Calibrator Graph (Fig. 2.29)

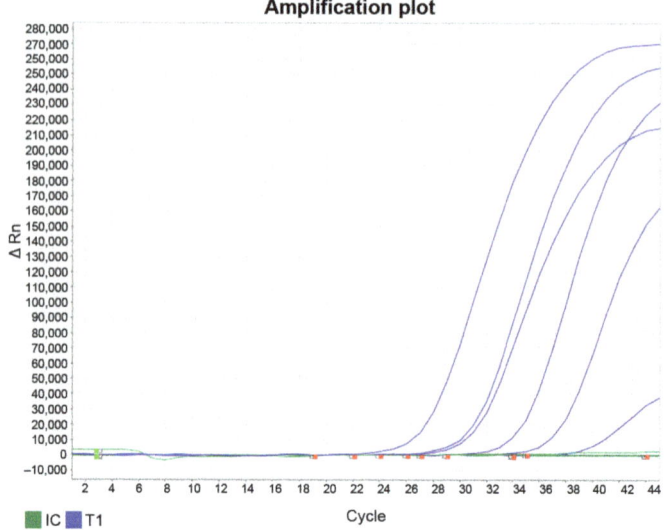

Fig. 2.29: Inconsistent spacing in calibrator graph.

Possible Causes
- Pipetting errors and Improper handling of reagents.
- Presence of inhibitors or contaminants.

Solutions
- Repeat the test. Ensure that the pipettes are calibrated.
- Ensure there are no inhibitors or contaminants in the reagents.
- Use no template control to check for presence of contamination.

APPLICATION OF MOLECULAR DIAGNOSTICS

Applications of Molecular Diagnostic Techniques.

Prenatal Tests

Conventional prenatal tests involve the analysis of the number and appearance of chromosomes (the karyotype). Noninvasive prenatal testing using fetal DNA in maternal plasma has been adopted due to the presence of cell-free DNA in plasma. The occurrence of mutation and inheritance patterns of diseases has given rise to prenatal diagnosis by use of direct or indirect methods of detection. In direct mutation analysis, detection is highly accurate whereas in indirect mutation analysis, accuracy is dependent on the distance between DNA marker and disease locus. This has been employed for chromosomal abnormalities such as Down syndrome.

Infectious Diseases

Molecular diagnostics are used to identify infectious diseases such as viral hepatitis, HIV, HPV, chlamydia, influenza virus and tuberculosis; or specific strains such as H1N1 virus, H3N2, Sars Cov 2 etc. FISH in combination with flow cytometry has been used for rapid culture independent detection of *Salmonella* species and in combination with PCR has been used for the accurate detection of Staphylococcus and Listeria.

Molecular diagnostics are also used to understand the specific strain of pathogens through the detection of drug resistance genes.

Cancer

Cancer is a change in the cellular processes that cause a tumor to grow out of control. Cancerous cells sometimes have mutations in oncogenes, such as KRAS and CTNNB1 (β-catenin). Analyzing the molecular signature of cancerous cells (the DNA and its levels of expression via mRNA) enables physicians to characterize the cancer and to choose the best therapy for their patients.

The incorporation of antibodies against specific protein marker molecules was developed and this could pave way for the development of multiplex assays that could measure many markers at a time. Other biomarkers expressed in excessive nature in cancerous cells relative to in healthy ones include micro-RNA molecules healthy ones. The development of molecular diagnostics by gliomas using next generation sequencing of a glioma-tailored gene panel has proved promising. Expression levels from a collection of DNA samples can be used in predicting cancer. This is due to the vast number of genes expression level.

DNA microarray with the help of multiresolution analysis tool, dual tree M-band wavelet transform (DTMBWT) for extraction at the 2nd level of decomposition and K-nearest neighbor (KNN) classifier, cancer classification into five different cancer datasets; Breast, colon, ovarian, CNS, and Leukemia with over 90% accuracy is now possible.

Drug Development

The utilization of DNA barcoding, microarray technology and sequencing for the elucidation of plant genetic diversity and conservation has proved promising in molecular biology. The newer trends utilized in DNA chips and barcoding have paved the way for a future with many different possibilities. This can assist to cure many different diseases and will also generate novel opportunities in medicinal drug delivery and targeting.

EVOLUTION OF PCR

The development of the polymerase chain reaction (PCR) has been a breakthrough in the scientific world. Over time, the technique has evolved beyond the confines of its simple initial design and has opened incredible avenues for researchers. Within 20 years of its discovery, this sensational technique became the basis for several molecular biology protocols and formed the foundation of the Human Genome Project.

The history of PCR technology, like all major developments in science, is marred by controversies, claims, and counterclaims, some of them still unresolved. This article seeks to chronicle the key developments leading to and after the invention of PCR.

In the year 1953, Watson and Crick discovered the double-helix structure of the DNA, showing that DNA has two strands with complementary bases running in opposite directions. More importantly, their report mulled over the possibility of a copying mechanism for DNA. Their double helix structure won them the Nobel Prize in 1962.

The first DNA polymerase was identified by Arthur Kornberg in 1957 during his studies on the DNA replication mechanism. This enzyme needed a primer to start copying the template and could create DNA only in one direction.

In 1971, Gobind Khorana, a Nobel Prize winner for his part in the Genetic Code discovery, and his team of researchers started working on DNA repair synthesis. This technique sought to simplify gene synthesis by using artificial primers and templates that help DNA polymerase to copy the desired gene segments.

Although this technique used DNA polymerase repeatedly, like PCR, it employed only a single primer template complex, and exponential amplification was not possible using this technique. Around the same time, Kjell Kleppe from Khorana's lab envisioned the use of a two-primer system which might help in desired DNA segment replication, forming an early precursor to PCR.

Research at Cetus Corporation

Cetus Corporation, a biotechnology company that will become home to most of the research leading to PCR, was founded in 1971. Kary Mullis of Cetus worked on oligonucleotides synthesis for use as probes, primers, and building blocks for various molecular biology techniques. Although he synthesized these oligos manually, he evaluated some automated synthesizer prototypes later on.

DNA Sequencing and the Advent of PCR

In the year 1977, Frederick Sanger identified a DNA sequencing method involving a DNA polymerase, a primer, and nucleotide precursors, for which he was awarded the Nobel Prize in 1980. Thus, by the year 1980, all components for PCR amplification were ready.

However, it was not until 1983 that to fix some issues in his research work, Mullis used Sanger's DNA sequencing method as a basis to devise a new technique. He added a second primer to the opposite strand and realized that repeated use of DNA polymerase will trigger a chain reaction that will amplify a specific DNA segment thus, discovering the PCR technology.

Analysis of PCR Products—Southern Blotting

Karry Mullis continued to test his idea, initially without thermal cycling but later with repeated thermal cycling. In 1984, Mullis along with the genetic mutation assay team at Cetus started working on experiments that show PCR's ability to amplify genomic DNA.

Although the amplification product was not evident in agarose gel electrophoresis initially, southern blotting confirmed the increase in quantity of the desired DNA segments.

The amplified DNA from PCR was successfully cloned and sequenced by the researchers, who applied for patent on PCR and its applications and got the patent approved in 1987. Meanwhile, the team used PCR for other applications by designing new primers and probes, which made the reaction more specific until the results were evident on agarose gel electrophoresis.

Taq DNA Polymerase

A major breakthrough in DNA polymerase came along in the year 1969, when Thomas Brock reported the isolation of *Thermus aquaticus*, a new species of thermophilic bacterium found in the hot springs of Yellowstone National Park. The DNA polymerase from this bacterium, called the Taq polymerase, could withstand very high temperatures, unlike other polymerases available at that point of time.

After a couple of failed attempts to isolate the Taq DNA polymerase, Susanne Stoffel and David Gelfand from Cetus finally isolated it in the fall of 1985, and Randy Saiki's experiments soon after proved that Taq polymerase is ideal for the PCR process. He went on to report the path breaking PCR technique to the scientific world in October 1985 and Mullis and his group published papers on PCR and its applications in leading science journals. A patent for PCR using Taq polymerase was issued in October 1990.

PerkinElmer and Cetus Develop PCR Machines

During the end of 1985, PerkinElmer and Cetus formed a joint venture to develop reagents and instruments for the PCR technique.

The manufacture of Taq-based PCR machines followed and the "AmpliTaq DNA Polymerase" was commercially available in November 1987.

PCR Applied to New Arenas

PCR was used to quantify the HIV in blood in the spring of 1985. By mid-1987, a viable test was available, and PCR was used to study the impact of antiviral drugs and also to screen donor blood samples for HIV. In October 1985, PCR was used to analyze sickle cell anemia, in its first clinical application.

Forensics scientist, Edward Blake joined hands with the FBI and Cetus researchers in 1986 to successfully use PCR for analysis of criminal evidence. But it was not until 1989 that highly sensitive DNA Fingerprinting tests were devised based on the PCR technique, making it an integral part of criminal investigations.

In 1987, DNA from a strand of human hair was amplified using PCR and this confirmed the ability of PCR to amplify DNA present in degraded samples part of forensic evidence.

Multiplex-PCR was described to analyze the meiotic recombination products in 1989. These single-copy amplifications later proved crucial for the study of DNA and genotyping.

Nobel Prize for Kary Mullis

Kary Mullis was awarded the Nobel Prize in Chemistry in October 1993, <10 years after the advent of PCR. In December 1989, Taq Polymerase was named "Molecule of the Year" by the journal Science. The Taq PCR paper later became the most cited publication in biology and PCR accounts for over 3% of all citations on PubMed.

Summary

The PCR technique as we know today was conceptualized and developed in the 1980s by Kary Mullis and his colleagues at Cetus Corporation. The isolation and purification of thermostable Taq polymerases led to the automation of the initially slow and laborious PCR technique and the development of programmable PCR thermal cyclers made it a widely used technique at many levels of biology and chemistry.

Although Mullis invented the PCR, its successful applications in several fields are a result of a lot of hard work by other Cetus researchers such as Henry Erlich. Also, there are challenges to the PCR patents held by Mullis based on early research works performed by Khorana et al. in the 1960s and 1970s.

Thanks to its extraordinary versatility, today, PCR is being used in diverse fields such as forensic science, environmental studies, food technology, and diagnostic medicine. The massive advancement over the years in our understanding of the genome of humans and several other species would not have been possible without the remarkable yet simple technique called PCR.

Conclusion

Molecular diagnostics are changing every aspect of biological sciences. However, for each of these technologies, the additions to health care costs must be weighed against the potential advantages of more rapid diagnostics. The carrying out of well-controlled outcome studies are necessary to demonstrate the efficacy of these technologies. Furthermore, the classifications of neoplastic diseases by newer molecular techniques are expected to soon complement the currently familiar histology-based classification systems.

JOURNEY OF RT PCR

PCR was invented over 38 years ago by Kary Mullis [Saiki, 1985], for which he received the Nobel Prize in Chemistry in 1993.

PCR is the innovation which allowed molecular biology to evolve to the current level. It has become a sensitive, specific, and reliable technique in life science research and more recently in routine human diagnostics.

When the PCR was invented the performing the test was so tedious and it could not be performed at normal laboratory setup and was restricted to research laboratory.

The extraction of the nucleic acid was one of the challenges and had to undergo different downstream processes from purification to further PCR under three different temperature heat baths for 40 cycles and was separated on gel electrophoresis for detection and gel doc system for analysis.

Later in 1992 the Real time PCR was invented where the PCR and detection system was integrated and minimize the resources to performing the test and allowed to use PCR in detection of microorganism and clinical diagnostics as well.

PCR has revolutionized over the past decade from a technically complicated method to a simple and easy to apply method. There is a wide variety of ready-to-use reagents available that allows those with some basic training and who master the skill of pipetting to perform a PCR. Enzymes and instruments have been continuously engineered to speed up the PCR process, so that a PCR can presently be performed in less than half an hour.

However, the simplicity of the method is its strength and weakness at the same time.

CURRENT CHALLENGES

Transportation and Storage

Despite of higher sensitivity and specificity the RT-PCR test does have some pitfalls that necessitate improvements in the way that reagents are stored. In India due to geographical diversity in temperature and wide geographical area maintaining $-20^{\circ}C$ and $-80^{\circ}C$ is quite difficult for the RT PCR Reagent storage and transportation.

Solution

Like other diagnostics kits of immunology and serology where the temperature requirement is 2–8° require less effort to store and transport the reagent. RT PCR kit should have the similar facility in order to increase its reach and make it accessible for laboratories on a large scale.

Optimal Uses of Reagent

Most of the commercially available RT-PCR reagents come in bigger pack size, for this reason diagnostic laboratories first accumulates samples than they run in a batch. This delay in testing reflects the sensitivity of the sample and degradation of viral nucleic acid in the sample.

Solution

The Ready to use Lyophilized single tube PCR mix is one of the solutions to optimal use of reagent. This single tube solution help laboratory to run the sample when the sample is requested for

PCR thereby enhancing the sensitivity of the test and reporting time of the laboratory.

Reagent Handling

Handling of Reagent in laboratory is one of the major challenges while performing molecular diagnostics test. It requires high expertise to handle the reagent due to its highly precise volume requirement. In diagnostics most of the sample are infectious, hazardous and can lead to contamination if mishandled.

Solution

A ready to use PCR mix and minimal pipetting step will lower down the potentially hazardousness and will prevent the contamination. The lyophilized master mix and precise uniform sample volume will minimize the need of highly expert technical person. The single tube will also inhibit the sample labeling error and mismatch of the sample due to manual error.

Clinical Sample Integrity

The molecular diagnostics tests are performed in bigger city and clinical sample are transported due to unavailability of resources to perform the molecular diagnostics because of low workload in tier II and tier III towns.

Solution

Decentralization of the laboratory is required to prevent the sample deterioration and result integrity. The ready to use PCR solution will enable the laboratory to perform the test with minimum resources and even with lower sample workload for better disease management in chronic diseases thus promoting better patient care.

Need of the Hour

Given the difficulties of the RT-PCR test, enormous efforts have been made to produce an easier, faster, and more convenient test capable of being used outside the laboratory environment. A simple and rapid test can reduce the sampling-to-result time (SRT) and encourage its wider application. The test procedure should require fewer steps and laboratory tools. A shorter SRT and easier manipulation of the sample will have some other benefits, including an increase in the test sensitivity.

Another invention which has made the test more convenient and quicker is where the pre-PCR step is combined with the PCR step itself. This reduction in the number of steps of the test offers some advantages:

1. A single step preparation of sample reduces the sampling to result time (SRT) and increases the potential of the test for wider application. A shorter SRT decreases the probability of disease transfer by individuals whose test results have yet to be determined.
2. A one-step preparation of the nucleic acid samples is much easier for potential users to learn how to use the test correctly.
3. During the extraction of nucleic acid from the sample, there is a risk of viral transmission from the samples to the laboratory staff, and cross-sample contamination due to unintentional errors in sample manipulation. A shorter and easier process of sample preparation can minimize the mentioned risks.

BIBLIOGRAPHY

1. Basics of Cell and Molecular Biology: Cell and Molecular Biology ISBN: 978-93-85740-54-1. Uttarakhand Open University Edition: 2017 Published by: Uttarakhand Open University, Haldwani, Nainital 263139.
2. Current applications and future trends of molecular diagnostics in clinical bacteriology. Analytical and Bioanalytical Chemistry (Eds.), Jan Weile & Cornelius Knabbe; 2009. 394:731-42.
3. Guidelines on Tuberculosis for India. Central TB Division Ministry of Health and Family Welfare, Government of India.
4. Microbiol. Food Microbiology. 8:2017.
5. Molecular Diagnostics and Therapeutics. Mol. Biosci., 17 July 2023 Sec. 10:2023.
6. National Essential Diagnostics List. Indian Council of Medical Research, Ansari Nagar, New Delhi-110029, India 2019.
7. Overcoming barriers to the uptake of molecular diagnostics NCRI's CM-Path Molecular Diagnostics Forum, 26th January 2018.
8. Sarkinfada F, Auwal IK, Manu, AY. Applications of molecular diagnostic techniques for infectious diseases. Department of Medical Microbiology and Parasitology, Faculty of Basic Clinical Sciences, College of Health Sciences, Bayero University, Kano Nigeria.

3 CHAPTER
Polymerase Chain Reaction in Clinical Diagnosis (Recapitulation in Brief)

EVOLUTION OF PCRs

While diagnostic modalities have evolved considerably from the beginning of the previous century, however, at a molecular level and that too related to genes and genetic sequencing has come into the arena since the end of the previous century. Nothing can be more specific to a pathogen other than the matter present with the nucleus viz., genes and their sequencing. This precisely is the crux of the PCR diagnostic technology.

What is a PCR?

The polymerase chain reaction (PCR) is a technique discovered by Dr. Kary B. Mullis in 1985 to synthesize multiple copies of a specific fragment of DNA from a template. The PCR reaction consists of cycling the DNA through three specific temperatures in a buffer solution consisting of the template, primers, nitrogenous bases and enzymes. It is capable of producing enormous amplification (i.e. identical copies) of a short DNA sequence from a single molecule of starter DNA. It is used to amplify a specific DNA (target) sequence lying between known positions (flanks) on a double-stranded (ds) DNA molecule.

The amplification process is mediated by oligonucleotide primers that, typically, are 20–30 nucleotides long. The primers are single stranded (ss) DNA that have sequences complementary to the flanking regions of the target sequence. Primers anneal to the flanking regions by complementary-base pairing (G≡C and A=T) using hydrogen bonding.

The amplified product is known as an amplicon.

Generally, PCR amplifies smallish DNA targets 100–1,000 base pairs (bp) long. (It is technically difficult to amplify targets >5,000 bp long.)

PCR has many applications in research, medicine and forensic science. PCR is a common and most indispensable technique used in medical laboratory and clinical laboratory research for a broad variety of applications including biomedical research and criminal forensics.

Polymerase chain reaction (PCR) is also extensively used in diagnosis of human diseases. Continuous enhancements to this filed have resulted in PCR becoming the gold standard techniques with very high sensitivity and high specificity in the diagnosis of various human diseases caused by,

- Viral, bacterial, fungal and parasitic pathogens
- Inherited disorders or genetic diseases
- Virally induced cancers, leukemia, lymphomas, and solid tumors to name a few.

With its ability to detect minute amounts of target DNA or RNA markers contained in tissues or biological fluids, PCR has improved the rapidity and accuracy of diagnosis, enhanced understanding of pathogenesis, and helped identify infectious causes for diseases previously considered idiopathic.

Principle of PCR (Fig. 3.1)

A PCR based diagnostic test starts with the process of target selection and primer design—identifying the sequence to be amplified and designing the primers accordingly. This critical step is responsible for the specificity of the PCR technique. The tremendous growth in genome sequence data coupled with advances in in-silico analysis have made this task comparatively more efficient than earlier. Primers are designed complementary to the template DNA. Two primers are used, one that binds to the sense strand, and another to the antisense strand. The primers are added, along with the DNA polymerase, dNTPs, magnesium chloride and DNA template strand.

Almost all the PCR methods are based on thermal cycling wherein the reactants in a PCR are exposed to repeated cycles of heating and cooling to allow different temperature dependent steps to proceed continuously at the specified temperatures. PCR comprises of two main reagents namely primers and DNA polymerase. Primers or oligonucleotides are short single stranded DNA fragments having complementary sequence to that of the target DNA strand. DNA polymerase is an enzyme that helps in the addition and extension of the new DNA strand. Almost all PCR applications employ a heat-stable DNA polymerase, known as Taq polymerase, an enzyme originally isolated from the thermophilic bacterium *Thermus aquaticus*. This enzyme is a heat stable enzyme. Apart from these two main components PCR also comprises of a PCR buffer, magnesium chloride and dNTPs (deoxyribonucleotide triphosphate).

One PCR cycle consists of three steps:
1. Denaturation
2. Annealing
3. Extension

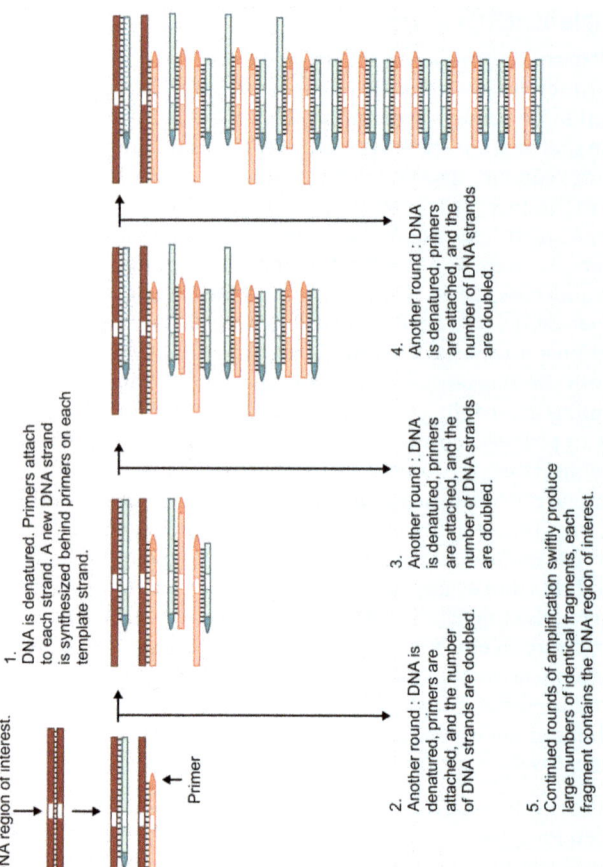

Fig. 3.1: Polymerase chain reaction.

Denaturation by Heat

Heat (usually >90°C) separates double-stranded DNA into two single strands, referred to as "denaturation". Since the hydrogen bonds linking the bases to one another are weak, they break at high temperatures, whereas the bonds between deoxyribose and phosphates, which are stronger covalent bonds, remain intact.

Annealing Primer Binding to Target

Primers are short, synthetic sequences of single stranded DNA typically consisting of 20–30 bases, with a biotin-labelled 5' end to aid in detection. They are specific for the target region of the organism. Two primers are included in the PCR, one for each of the complementary single DNA strands that was produced during denaturation. The beginning of the DNA target sequence of interest is marked by the primers that anneal (bind) to the complementary sequence.

Annealing temperature: Annealing usually takes place between 40°C and 65°C, depending on the length and base sequence of the primers. This allows the primers to anneal to the target sequence with high specificity.

Extension

Once the primers anneal to the complementary DNA sequences, the temperature is raised to approximately 72°C and the enzyme Taq DNA polymerase is used to replicate the DNA strands. Taq DNA polymerase is a recombinant thermostable DNA polymerase from the organism *Thermus aquaticus* and, unlike normal polymerase enzymes is active at high temperatures.

Taq DNA polymerase begins the synthesis process at the region marked by the primers. It synthesizes new double-stranded DNA molecules, both identical to the original double stranded target DNA region, by facilitating the binding and joining of the complementary nucleotides that are free in solution (dNTPs). Extension always begins at the 3' end of the primer making a double strand out of each of the two single strands. Taq DNA polymerase synthesizes exclusively in the 5' to 3' direction. Therefore, free nucleotides in the solution are only added to the 3' end of the primers constructing the complementary strand of the targeted DNA sequence.

Following primer extension, the mixture is heated (again at 90–95°C) to denature the molecules and separate the strands and the cycle repeated.

Each new strand then acts as a template for the next cycle of synthesis. Thus amplification proceeds at an exponential (logarithmic) rate, i.e., amount of DNA produced doubles at each cycle. 30–35 cycles of amplification can yield around 1 µg DNA of 2,000 bp length from 10^{-6} µg original template DNA. This is a million-fold amplification.

Initially, the 3 different stages at 3 different temperatures were carried out in separate water baths but nowadays, a thermal cycler is used (a machine that automatically changes the temperature at the correct time for each of the stages and can be programed to carry out a set number of cycles).

A typical thermal cycle might be as follows: Heat denaturation at 94° for 20 seconds primer annealing at 55° for 20 seconds primer extension at 72° for 30 seconds total time for one cycle = approx. 4 minutes.

- ❖ **DNA is denatured:** Primers attach to each strand. A new DNA strand is synthesized behind primers on each template strand.

- **Another round:** DNA is denatured, primers are attached, and the number of DNA strands are doubled.
- **Another round:** DNA is denatured, primers are attached, and the number of DNA strands are doubled.
- **Another round:** DNA is denatured, primers are attached, and the number of DNA strands are doubled.
- **Continued rounds:** Continued rounds of amplification swiftly produce large numbers of identical fragments. Each fragment contains the DNA region of interest.

Types of PCR

RT-PCR

This is reverse transcriptase-PCR and is a two-stage procedure used for the amplification of RNA. The first stage employs an enzyme called reverse transcriptase, which synthesizes a DNA strand complementary to the RNA of interest by using one of the PCR primer as its primer. The complementary DNA is then used in the second stage as the starting material for PCR amplification by a conventional thermostable DNA polymerase.

Nested PCR

It is a PCR done in two steps, a primary PCR reaction and a nested reaction. The primary (or first) reaction uses a set of primers to generate a product that serves as the template for the nested (or second) reaction. The nested reaction uses a set of PCR primers specific for a region within the amplified product from the first reaction. Therefore, the nested reaction often serves as a confirmation for the specificity of the PCR products amplified in the primary reaction.

Real-Time PCR (Fig. 3.2)

Combines PCR amplification and detection into a single step. The basic principle of real-time quantitative PCR is the detection of target sequences using a fluorogenic 5' nuclease assay (often called 'TaqMan').

Real-time or Quantitative PCR (qPCR) is used for the amplification of DNA in a linear manner in order to quantify absolute or relative amounts of target sequence in a sample. With the help of a fluorescent reporter, the amount of generated DNA can be measured. In qPCR, DNA amplification is monitored at each cycle

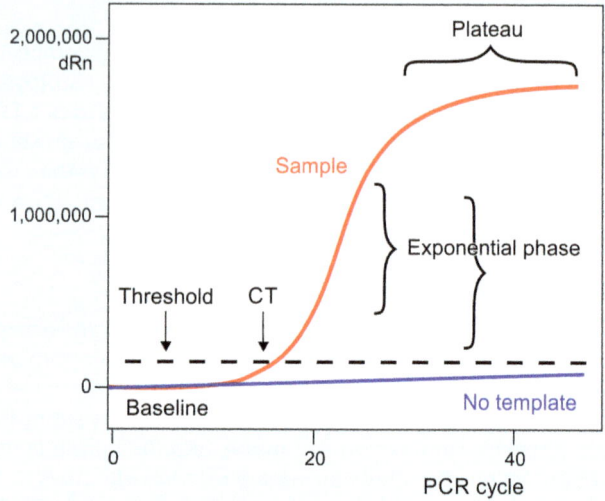

Fig. 3.2: Depiction of real time PCR plot.
Courtesy: NPTEL (National programme on technology enhanced learning)]

of PCR. When the DNA is getting amplified logarithmically at each cycle, the amount of fluorescence increases over the basal level. The thermal cycle at which the signal exceeds the fluorescence detection threshold is known as the **Threshold cycle** (C_T) or crossing point. A standard curve of log concentration against C_T can be made by making use of multiple dilutions of a known amount of standard DNA. The quantity of DNA or cDNA in an unknown sample can thus be determined from its C_T value.

Different chemistries are used for detection by q PCR:

❖ Use of an intercalating dye like the SYBR® Green I dye **(Fig. 3.3)** which incorporates between the base pairs of DNA. This detection method is suitable when the PCR reaction

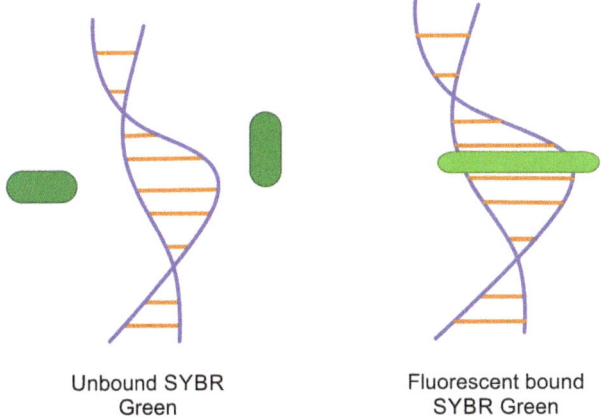

Unbound SYBR Green

Fluorescent bound SYBR Green

Fig. 3.3: Showing mechanism of attachment of SYBR green dye to DNA.
Courtesy: NPTEL (National programme on technology enhanced learning)]

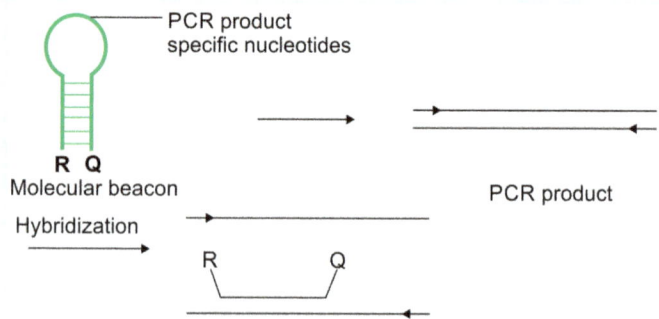

Fig. 3.4: Molecular beacon based PCR detection.
Courtesy: NPTEL (National programme on technology enhanced learning)]

generates a specific product, as the dye is capable of intercalating into any double-stranded DNA product.

- Use of primer or short oligonucleotide specific to the target of interest, as in TaqMan® probes, Molecular beacons™, **(Fig. 3.4)** or scorpion primers. In case of molecular beacons, they are labeled with a fluorescent dye or quencher and do not exhibit any significant fluorescence in the free, unhybridized condition. But upon binding to the template, the probe becomes fluorescent as the quencher gets distanced from the fluorescent reporter. The amount of PCR product amplified is directly proportional to the amount of fluorescence.
- **TaqMan probe based detection (Fig. 3.5):** While in the case of TaqMan® probes, fluorescence occurs when the dye is clipped from the probe during the polymerase extension.

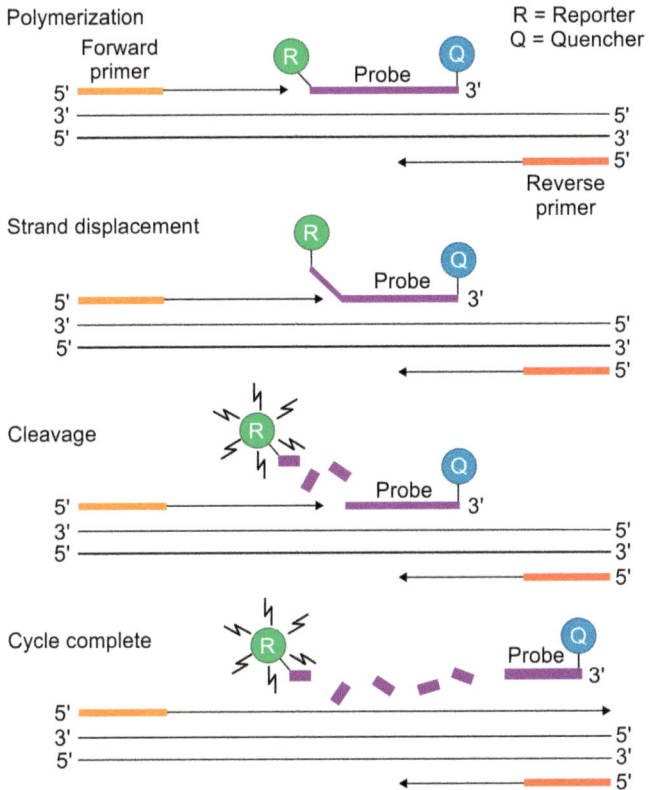

Fig. 3.5: TaqMan probe-based PCR detection.

- **Ligation-mediated PCR**: It uses small DNA oligonucleotide 'linkers' (or adaptors) that are first ligated to fragments of the target DNA.
- **Methylation-specific PCR** (MSP): It is used to identify patterns of DNA methylation at cytosine-guanine (CpG) islands in genomic DNA.
- **Multiplex-PCR**: It uses several pairs of primers annealing to different target sequences.
- **Variable number of tandem repeats (VNTR) PCR**: It targets areas of the genome that exhibit length variation.
- **Asymmetric PCR**: It preferentially amplifies one strand of the target DNA.
- **Nested PCR**: It is used to increase the specificity of DNA amplification. Two sets of primers are used in two successive reactions. In the first PCR, one pair of primers is used to generate DNA products, which may contain products amplified from non-target areas. The products from the first PCR are then used as template in a second PCR, using one ('hemi-nesting') or two different primers whose binding sites are located (nested) within the first set, thus increasing specificity.

The advantages of this system include high reproducibility, the capability of handling large numbers of samples, the potential for quantitative results, and decreased turnaround time. The disadvantages include high instrument cost and the requirement for technical proficiency.

Multiplex PCR

It is a PCR designed to detect more than one target sequence in a single PCR reaction. The assay uses two or more sets of primers.

Each set of primers is specific for a different target sequence. The assay is most commonly used for simultaneous detection of multiple viral genes and differentiation of genotypes or subtypes of related microorganisms.

Differential PCR

Differential PCR can sometimes be used to distinguish closely related targets. Differential PCR is done either in a multiplex format using two or more sets of primers or by running two separate PCR assays.

APPLICATIONS OF PCR

PCR technique has vast applications. It can be used for DNA cloning application for sequencing, gene cloning and manipulation, gene mutagenesis; construction of DNA-based phylogenies, functional analysis of genes, diagnosis and monitoring of hereditary diseases, amplification of ancient DNA, analysis of genetic fingerprints for DNA profiling (for example, in forensic science and parentage testing), and finally it has a huge impact in the detection of pathogens for infectious disease diagnosis.

ADVANTAGES OF PCR OVER CONVENTIONAL TECHNIQUES

- Quick, accurate, more sensitive and specific
- Has fast turnaround time as compared to other tests such as culture
- Has more wider application such as detecting infectious diseases, genetic testing, forensics, drug resistance, and tumor marker detection and monitoring.

LIMITATIONS/DIFFICULTIES

Technique Related Limitations

While a very powerful technique, PCR can also be very tricky. The polymerase reaction is very sensitive to the levels of divalent cations (especially Mg^{2+}) and nucleotides, and the conditions for each particular application must be worked out. Primer design is extremely important for effective amplification. The primers for the reaction must be very specific for the template to be amplified. Cross reactivity with non-target DNA sequences results in nonspecific amplification of DNA. Also, the primers must not be capable of annealing to themselves or each other, as this will result in the very efficient amplification of short nonsense DNAs. The reaction is limited in the size of the DNAs to be amplified (i.e., the distance apart that the primers can be placed). The most efficient amplification is in the 300–1,000 bp range, however, amplification of products up to 4 Kb has been reported. Also, Taq polymerase has been reported to make frequent mismatch mistakes when incorporating new bases into a strand.

PCR reagents are very sensitive to heat and are stored at temperatures between –20°C and 80°C and cannot be subjected to multiple freeze thaw cycles. Laboratories running PCR are typically equipped with good sample storage facilities and skilled technicians.

The most important consideration in PCR is contamination. If the sample that is being tested has even the smallest contamination with DNA from the target, the reaction could amplify this DNA and report a falsely positive identification. For example, if a technician in a crime lab sets up a test reaction (with blood from the crime scene) after setting up a positive control reaction (with blood from the suspect) cross contamination between the samples could result in an erroneous incrimination, even if the technician changed pipette tips between samples. A few blood cells could volatilize in the pipette, stick to the plastic of the pipette, and then get ejected into the test sample. The powerful amplification of PCR may be able to detect this cross contamination of samples. Modern labs take account of this fact and devote tremendous effort to avoiding this problem, while strictly following good laboratory practices to ensure accurate reporting of results.

Because of the high capex and opex involved in the above, clinical diagnostic applications of PCR have been highly centralized and limited to large hospitals and laboratories having specialized infrastructure and resources. Samples hence have to be transported to these centralized facilities, maintaining a cold chain. These and the need for batch testing often lead to long turnaround time for results, thus severely limiting the clinical value of the test.

New innovations in recent times have come up with solutions that enable decentralization of PCR testing by reducing/eliminating dependence on laboratory infrastructure and skilled manpower and bringing PCR testing closer to the patient.

Point of Care PCR for Clinical Diagnosis

In order to cater to the need for PCR based diagnosis in distributed settings, PCR devices are becoming smaller, simpler, more accurate, and easy to handle. The introduction of GeneXpert by Cepheid, Sunnyvale, California paved the way for more affordable and less complicated real time PCR testing. However, infrastructure dependence resulted in this platform being restricted to district level settings.

CHAPTER 4

Practical Aspects/Actual Working on Systems

AMPLICHAIN™

INTRODUCTION

Real-time PCR quantitative PCR, qPCR is now a well-established method for the detection, quantification, and typing of different microbial agents in the areas of clinical and veterinary diagnostics and food safety. Although the concept of PCR is relatively simple, there are specific issues in qPCR that users of this technology must bear in mind. These include the use of correct terminology and definitions, understanding of the principle of PCR, difficulties with interpretation and presentation of data, the limitations of qPCR in different areas of microbial diagnostics and parameters important for the description of qPCR performance however, it is our hope that this basic guide will help to orient beginners and users of qPCR in the use of this powerful technique.

CURRENT CHALLENGE IN PERFORMING REAL-TIME PCR SYSTEM

Sample Collection and Transportation

Existing molecular tests based on polymerase chain reaction (PCR), though sensitive but still take time as specimens are often sent to distant referral laboratories. The expense and infrastructure involved in PCR testing establishes a barrier to implementation into routine laboratory. Identification of multidrug resistance in this system is a tedious and time-consuming process. Quick and affordable diagnosis is critical to prevent major infectious disease.

Sample Extraction and Purification

The extraction and purification of nucleic acids from a clinical specimen is necessary. It frees the extracted nucleic acids from potential PCR inhibitors and cell debris. If PCR inhibitors are present in nucleic acid sample, it will give false negative result.

Common challenges in nucleic acid extraction include a limited number of technical staff, high staff turnover, and the use of different processing protocols across various commercial kits. These factors often lead to variability in the purity and yield of extraction results, even for the same sample.

Additionally, achieving repeatability and reproducibility of results between trained technical staff and across different laboratories is a significant concern. Each laboratory strives to mitigate this variance caused by human factors.

By reducing or minimizing human intervention during testing, more accurate and efficient results can be obtained. Automated extraction platforms play a crucial role in this regard, enhancing the precision and effectiveness of diagnostic processes. The implementation of automated nucleic acid extraction technology is key to improving the reliability and consistency of diagnostics.

Special Infrastructure Requirement

To perform a PCR run there is a huge laboratory infrastructure requirement that need to establish. Starting from clean room to various separate room for preparation of reagent, buffer, and its component. The lack of technical expertise leads to misguided outcome.

Reporting the Results

Before producing the final report in clinical diagnosis real-time PCR required a lot of interpretation. The major challenge into this interpretation is due to involvement of multiple venders. The highly technical expertise is required to come on conclusion. Sometime the test needs to be repeated to ruled out possible reason results delay in reporting time.

WHAT IS THE NEED?

There has been an urgent need to develop cost effective molecular test system that can be used within the low infrastructure setup.

The system should be cost-effective, but should offer ease of use, diagnostic sensitivity. Such a system will enhance the efforts to treat diseases before they spread and cause irreversible damage to the patient's health and safety. This kind of system is an ideal candidate for wide-scale use among the peripheral laboratories.

There are recent examples of the development in the field of molecular diagnostics as a point of care system based on automated real-time PCR that simultaneously detects both *Mycobacterium tuberculosis* complex (MTBC) and rifampicin (RIF) resistance in <2 hours. Such a system is often limited to laboratories with a controlled environment and low throughput.

"There is an urgent need for cost-effective molecular test system that offers promised sensitivity, specificity. The system should have low to medium throughput and should work in low-infrastructure setup so that it can screen the population of the community and

suffice the need of wider population and could save thousands of lives."

OBJECTIVE AND PURPOSE

Our primary objective is to suffice the above need and develop a PCR based molecular system which can run in a low infrastructure setup laboratory and offers promised sensitivity, specificity with a medium throughput.

The system should be capable of serving up to community health centre (CHC) in which primary objective is to diagnose the first point of contact with molecular testing and will help to overcome the limitation of traditional diagnosis.

The system should be flexible in terms of installation needs and user friendly as it should not require any special training to operate.

INTRODUCTION OF AMPLICHAIN INSTRUMENT AND REAGENT

Tulip Diagnostics has developed **Amplichain^{TM} PCR station**—Real-Time PCR-based automated system, which comprises of:

- **Amplichain^{TM} Ex32**: Automated magnetic beads based nucleic acid extraction system
- **Amplichain^{TM} qPCR:** A real-time quantitative PCR instrument.

Both the systems will be supported by Amplichain^{TM} reagents for magnetic beads based extraction and Amplichain^{TM} PCR reagent packs. Amplichain PCR station will also include all the accessories like Pipettes, stands to hold elute collection tubes and PCR tubes which will be required in workflow.

The amplichain system will support single tests and batch testing up to 16 tests. A batch can be performed in <2 hour of time span.

The Amplichain PCR reagents will be in two different formats:
1. **Amplichain™ MonoTest:** All MonoTest packs will have individual PCR tubes prefilled with lyophilized master mix. This will allow user to use individual test without affecting integrity and shelf life of the remaining reagent.
2. **Amplichain™ MultiTest:** All MultiTest packs will have vials filled with lyophilized master mix. Each vial will suffice 24 tests.

The reagents and instruments can be operated at temperatures ranging from 15 to 45°C. Storage temperature for amplichain PCR reagents will be from 2 to 8°C with stability of one year.

The workflow of amplichain PCR station is designed to have only two steps user intervention, this will increase result integrity and turnaround time.

Principle

Amplichain is based on **real-time PCR TaqMan probe-based** principle where the system will work in following steps from patient specimen collection to result.

- ❖ **Patient sample collection and sample preparation:** To perform the molecular test in clinical diagnostics it is very important to collect and process appropriate samples in line with specific disease. The common sample type is serum, blood, plasma, swab (specimen in specific media). These samples can be directly processed for nucleic acid extraction and purification. Apart from these the sample needs to be processed for homogenization.
- ❖ **For other samples:**
    - Check if the specimen is pipettable. If not, add 1 drop of liquefaction buffer, amplichain sample pretreatment kit to

the specimen (if specimen is frozen allow it to reach room temperature first).
- Allow the reagent to hydrate the sample by swirling gently. Incubate at room temperature for 5 minutes and transfer 500 μL of the sample into it using the graduated transfer pipette provided.

Operating Instructions for Amplichain Ex-32 (Fig. 4.1)

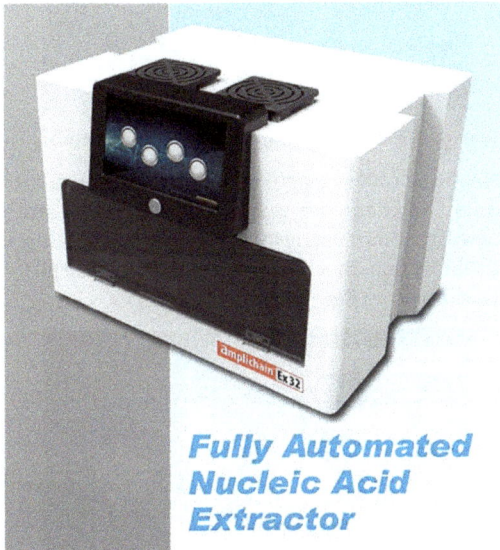

Fig. 4.1: Fully automated nucleic acid extractor.

Initializing the Instrument (Fig. 4.2)

Switch "ON" the power supply of the instrument. The display appears below.

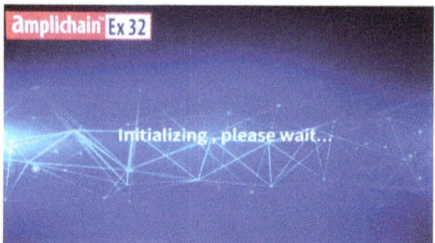

Fig. 4.2: Display at initializing the instrument.

Initialization process is activated. In the initialization process the instrument magnetic rod, magnetic cover holder and the plate rack holder will start initializing to their respective homing positions.

After initialization, the display automatically will go to the next page as shown below **(Fig. 4.3)**.

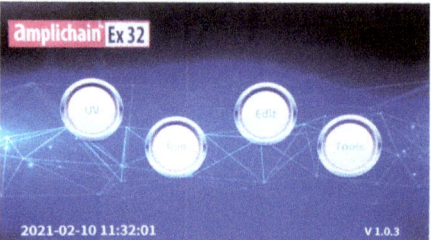

Fig. 4.3: Screen-post initialization.

Running Amplichain Universal Kit

- Open the **amplichain universal** kit
- Remove all the components out (i.e., B1, B2, B3, B4, B5)
- Prepare the reagents, i.e., add extra ethanol in the provided reagents.

Reagents	Contents/Labels	Volume of ethanol to be added
B1	Lysis/binding buffer	25 mL
B3	Wash buffer A	15 mL
B4	Wash buffer B	35 mL

Note: B1, B3 and B4 are supplied as concentrate. Before using it for the first time, add the recommended volume of ethanol as indicated above and on the respective bottles.

Please tick mark the check box provided on the label after addition of ethanol.

- Use this prepared reagent for further processing.
- In well 1 add 600 µL of B1 and 300 µL of sample
- In well 2 add 100 µL of ethanol and 15 µL of B2
- In well 3 add 600 µL of B3 (wash buffer A)
- In well 4 add 600 µL of B4 (wash buffer B)
- Keep well no. 5 empty.
- In well no. 6 add 100 µL of B5 (elution buffer)

Loading Deep Well Plate (Fig. 4.4)

- Once the plate is ready to load into the instrument, load the magnetic rod cover.
- Load the prepared deep well plate as shown below image.

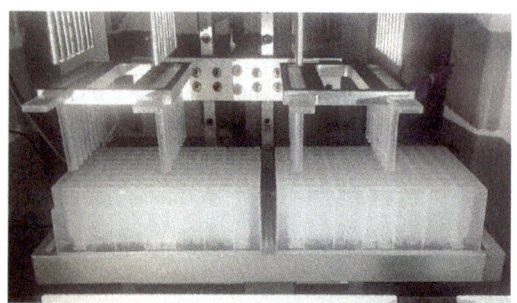

Fig. 4.4: Deep well plate.

- Select the RUN menu from the display **(Fig. 4.5).**

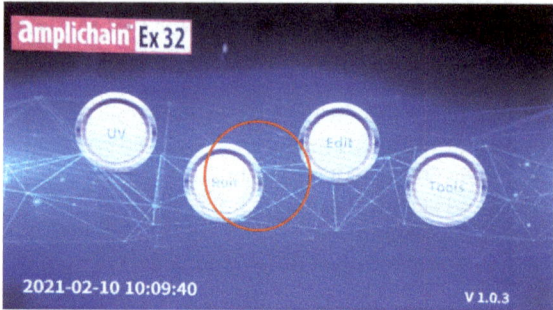

Fig. 4.5: RUN menu from the display.

- Select the desired program and touch on **OK** button on display **(Fig. 4.6).**

Chapter 4: Practical Aspects/Actual Working on Systems

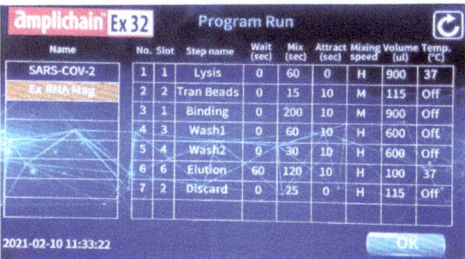

Fig. 4.6: Screen to select desired program.

❖ On display touch on **PLAY** option, the process will start **(Fig. 4.7).**

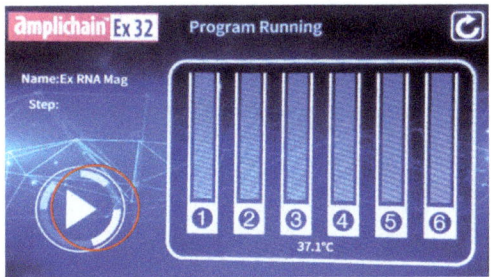

Fig. 4.7: Dispay of touch to play.

❖ After the completion of the program the elute buffer will be having the extracted RNA/DNA.
Note: Similarly, we have to perform the test for other parameters. (Please refer to reagent pack insert for test procedure).

Running the Test Parameter from Individuals Test Cartridges (Fig. 4.8)

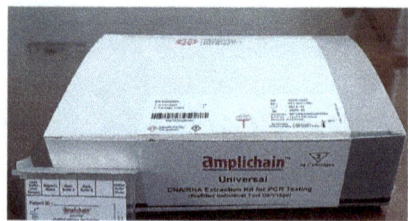

Fig. 4.8: Amplichain universal prefilled cartridges.

- ❖ Amplichain universal prefilled cartridges is designed to perform individual as well up to 8 test from clinical sample.
- ❖ Transfer the sample into the lysis chamber of amplichain universal cartridge for nucleic acid extraction **(Fig. 4.9)**.

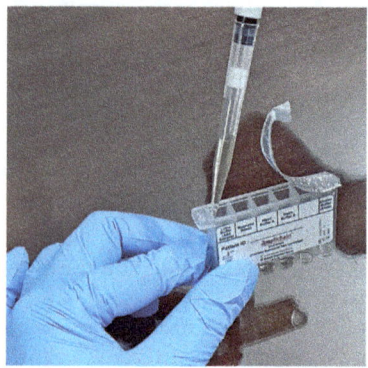

Fig. 4.9: Transferring sample to the amplichain universal prefilled cartridge.

- After lysis, this pretreatment tube is transferred to **Amplichain Ex 32** for nucleic acid extraction individual cartridges holder **(Fig. 4.10)**

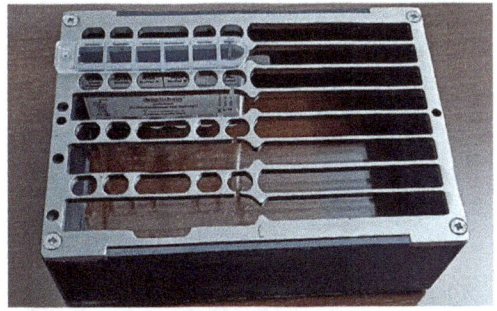

Fig. 4.10: Individual cartridges holder with prefilled cartridges.

- Once the extraction process is completed the extracted DNA material needs to be transferred to an Elute collection tube, which will be used for further investigation.
- The lysed sample can also be transported to the installed laboratory setup from primary health care center or from sub rural hospital.

Step 2: Setting up RT PCR System (Amplichain qPCR) (Fig. 4.11)

Amplichain qPCR is an automated qRT PCR system where real-time PCR and detection are performed simultaneously.

Amplichain qPCR having user defined login software where all the programs are preloaded to run the PCR test. Total 16 number of tests can be run in the system simultaneously.

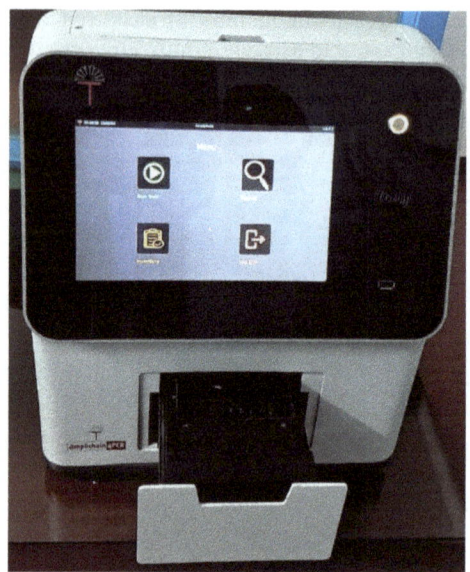

Fig. 4.11: Amplichain qPCR.

Procedure to Load the Test in Amplichain qPCR

❖ 10 μL of Extracted DNA from elute collection tube is added to the Amplichain™ disease specific PCR tube **(Fig. 4.12)** containing lyophilized master mix, which is provided with Amplichain™ PCR kit **(Figs. 4.13 and 4.14).**

Chapter 4: Practical Aspects/Actual Working on Systems

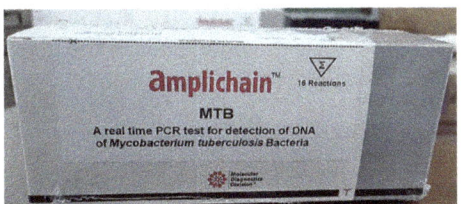

Fig. 4.12: Disease specific PCR tube.

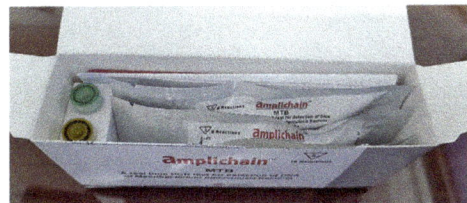

Fig. 4.13: Amplichain MTB PCR reagennt.

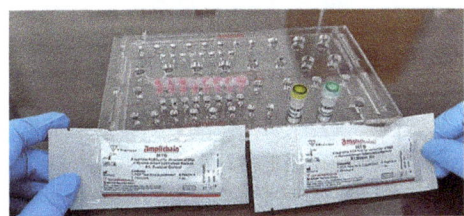

Fig. 4.14: Amplichain MTB PCR reagent in lyopilised pcr strip.

- **Reconstitution of PCR reagent (Fig. 4.15):** As the PCR tube is lyophilized before addition of elute in the tube it needs to be reconstituted with 10 µL reconstitution buffer provided in the PCR kit.

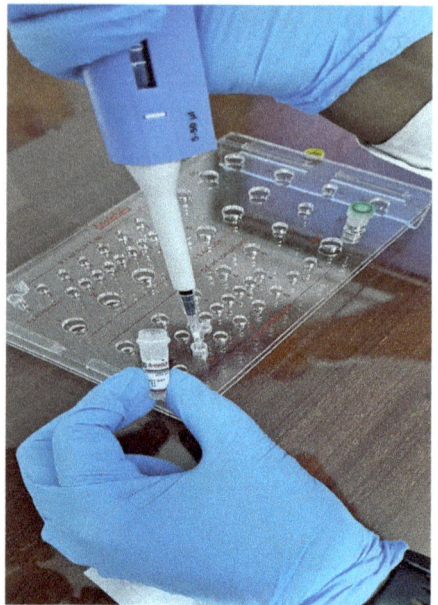

Fig. 4.15: Reconstitution of PCR tube with reconstitution buffer.

- **Addition of 10 µL od extracted nucleic acid (Fig. 4.16):** The extracted nucleic acid which were collected in the elute collection tube, 10 µL to be added in the reconstituted PCR tube.

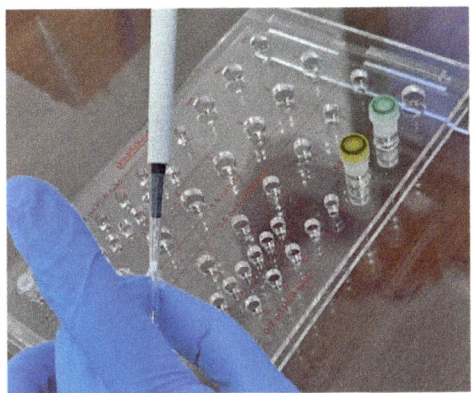

Fig. 4.16: Addition of template in PCR tube.

Set of Amplichain qPCR Test Run (Fig. 4.17)

- Login to the instrument with user defined login and password.

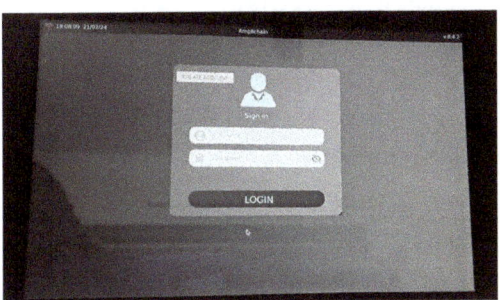

Fig. 4.17: Amplichain qPCR login window.

- Amplichain qPCR allow users to create a unique login to perform the test. The laboratory data will be more secure and authentic with this feature.
- **Running the test:** Click on RUN button to perform the test. **(Fig. 4.18)**

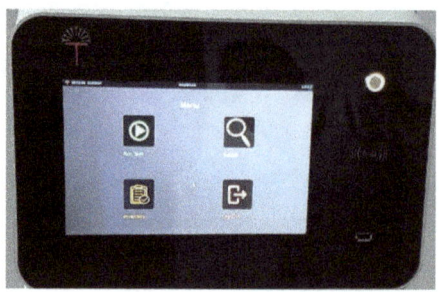

Fig. 4.18: Window after login page.

- Select number of well and patient detail respective to the corresponding well **(Fig. 4.19)**.

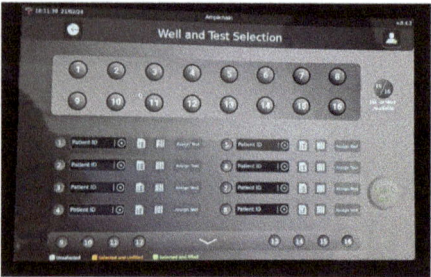

Fig. 4.19: Well selection and patient ID detail.

❖ The patient detail need to be fill with Patient ID, Name, Age, Sex, Sample Type and assign the test in tab of Assign Tab **(Fig. 4.20)**

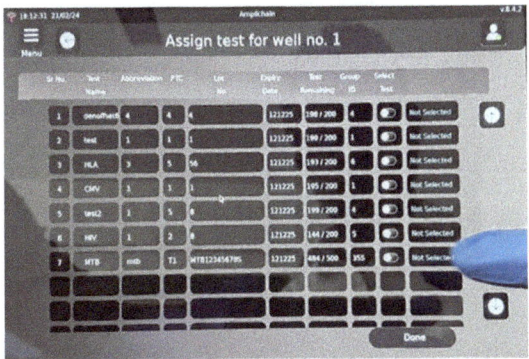

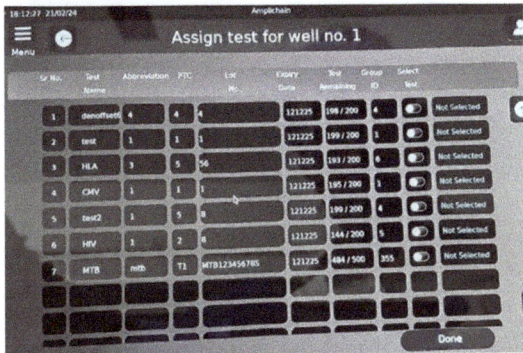

Fig. 4.20: Assigning of test for the selected well.

Chapter 4: Practical Aspects/Actual Working on Systems

- Verify the PCR tube **(Fig. 4.21)** with their unique disease specific PCR test code (PTC) mention in the PCR tube and position of the PCR tube in well.

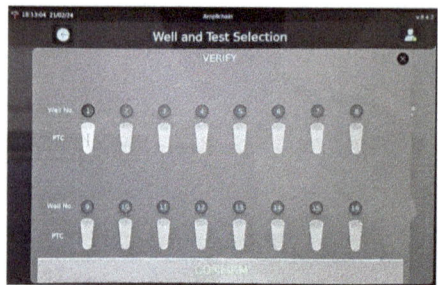

Fig. 4.21: Confirmation window for PCR tube.

- Close the gate of instrument and start the test **(Figs. 4.22 and 4.23)**

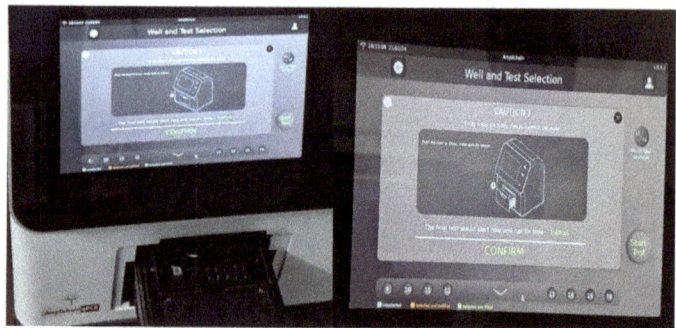

Fig. 4.22: Loading position of well and start button for PCR run.

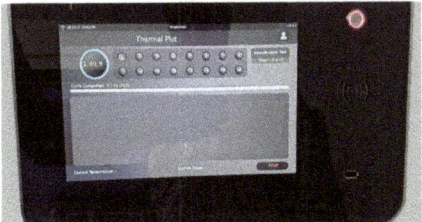

Fig. 4.23: Running of the test parameter.

Result

After completion of the test optical plot and result can be seen by click view optical curve and result **(Fig. 4.24)**

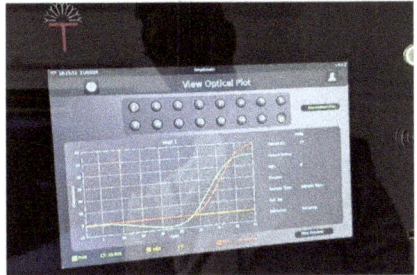

Fig. 4.24: Optical view and result window of qPCR instrument.

To run the RIF resistance for positive samples, the same elute collection tube containing extracted DNA can be used along with amplichain MTB RIF PCR tube containing lyophilized master mix.

The reagent system, amplification detection kit is based on TaqMan-based real-time PCR technique for amplification of DNA and fluorescence detection.

The TaqMan probes for the target gene are labeled with FAM and CY5 for target specific signal. The assay includes housekeeping gene as internal control to monitor the process from sample collection, nucleic acid extraction to fluorescence detection. The IC probe is labeled with HEX/VIC fluorescent dye to differentiate its fluorescent signal from target.

Specification

Amplichain™ Ex 32: Automated magnetic beads based nucleic acid extraction system.
- A low to medium throughput device which can extract 1–32 samples in 25 minutes.
- Small footprint—bench top design can be installed at any small laboratory set up.
- Magnetic beads based extraction promises highly sensitive and pure DNA extraction.
- Compatible with various type of samples.
- Preprogramed software, user only need to select the number of samples and start.
- Simple operation with operational integrity.
- UPS and mains operated which run on 220 V AC with operating temperature 15 to 45°C.

Amplichain™ qPCR: A real-time quantitative RT PCR instrument
- A low to medium throughput device which can perform 1–16 sample at one run which takes 1 to 2 hour time.
- Small footprint—bench top design can be installed at any small laboratory set up.
- TaqMan based chemistry proves highly specific and sensitivity technique.
- RFID card based operation for loading reagents, offers hazel free programming and minimum user intervention.

- Option of using amplichain reagents other than MTB.
- User friendly software operation.
- UPS and mains operated which run on 220 V AC with operating temperature 15 to 45°C.

Amplichain Reagents

- Room temperature stable reagent.
- Lyophilized master mix enhances the stability.
- MonoTest and MultiTest reagent kits.
- Target genes for high sensitivity and specificity.
- Housekeeping gene as internal control for process validation.
- One year expiry with storage between 2 and 8°C.

Parameter

The amplichain disease specific having multiple parameter for infectious and noninfectious.

Like

Amplichain^{TM} MTB

Amplichain^{TM} Dengue

Amplichain^{TM} Chikungunya

Amplichain^{TM} HPV 16 and18

Amplichain^{TM} HLAB27

Amplichain^{TM} Malaria Pf and Pv

Amplichain^{TM} CMV

Amplichain^{TM} universal magnetic beads

Conclusion

In conclusion, amplichain is independent of the user's skills, and routine staff with minimal training can use the test. It has a shorter turnaround time<2 hour. The amplichain platform can be installed at low level infrastructure like community health centre (CHC). In 8 hours of duration maximum 128 sample can be run. The system is inbuilt with enhanced user-friendly user interface and data of patient can be also uploaded on cloud server via internet.

5
CHAPTER
Commercially Available– Kits of an Open System

INNOVATIVE IDEAS SIMPLIFYING MOLECULAR DIAGNOSTICS

*Tulip has always led the way in developing "better testing systems for better diagnostics". Now with amplichain range of products we are stepping into molecular diagnostics. We understand the day-to-day challenges faced by molecular diagnostic laboratories which makes this technology complicated for all to use. Amplichain range of products is the result of our **Innovative Approach to Simplify Molecular Diagnostics.***

AMPLICHAIN

Molecular diagnostics has been the domain of large central laboratories where the high- end capital investment and molecular expert were required. The access to this technology was limited before the onset of SARS-CoV-2 virus. Now the infrastructure for molecular diagnostics has reached to various place but despite of available infrastructure, the technology is still not accessible to all. This is due to the present limitations which is creating challenges in using this technology.

The major challenges with present molecular diagnostics reagents and testing system are:

Centralized Testing

- Centralized testing forces sample transportation.
- Present reagent system forces batch testing.

Compromise on Sample Integrity and Delay in Test Report

Reagent Storage

- Need special refrigerator to maintain <-20°C.
- Reagents need to be aliquoted with limited freeze-thaw cycles.

Compromise on Reagent Sensitivity and Specificity

Larger Pack Size

- Need Capital Investment to procure the kit.
- Storage and usage require regular freeze thaw.

Incomplete Kit Utilization and Loss of Reagent Stability

Multiple Extraction Reagents

Separate reagents for DNA, RNA and different types of samples like sputum, blood etc.

Need to Maintain Multiple Kits

It is evident that molecular diagnostics is going to be the future of diagnostics but today we need to decentralize and simplify the molecular diagnostics testing.

AMPLICHAIN

SIMPLIFYING MOLECULAR DIAGNOSTICS

Amplichain range of products includes solutions for molecular diagnostics from nucleic acid extraction to real time PCR.

Highlights of amplichain reagents are lyophilised and monotest Master mix

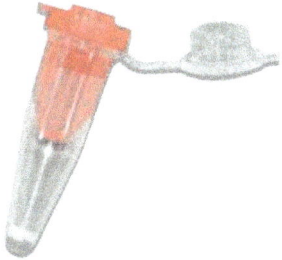

- Master mix is lyophilized and prefilled in PCR tube for single test with storage at 2-8°C.
- Convenient storage and transportation
- No batch testing
- Maintained reagent stability

Smaller Pack Size

The amplichain reagent are available in mono test 16 test and bulk test 48 test.
- Easy to use and store
- Ideal for special tests

User Friendly

Single test and single step with simple procedure
- Common step for all the test reagents
- Easy to perform and reduces pipetting error

Open and Optimized

- Amplichain reagents are open and optimized with three most widely used open RT PCR Instruments
- Validated protocols

Endogenous Control

The endogenous control gene is inbuilt in each test for validation of process from extraction to PCR Result.
- Complete process control
- Validates sample integrity

UNIVERSAL NUCLEIC ACID EXTRACTION KIT

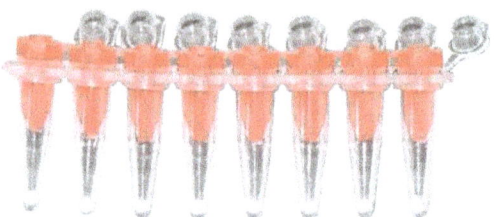

- Magnetic beads based single kit for all type of samples
- Available in manual and automated platform

SIMPLIFYING MOLECULAR DIAGNOSTICS

Amplichain® Product Range

Nucleic Acid Extraction

Amplichain Universal—DNA/RNA extraction kit for PCR testing (magnetic bead method)

Real Time PCR Kits

- **Amplichain MTB:** A real time PCR test for detection of DNA of *Mycobacterium tuberculosis* bacteria
- **Amplichain malaria Pf and Pv:** A real time PCR duplex test for detection of DNA of malaria Pf and Pv parasites
- **Amplichain CMV:** A real time PCR test for detection of DNA of CMV
- **Amplichain dengue and ChikV:** A real time PCR duplex test for detection of RNA of dengue and chikungunya virus
- **Amplichain dengue:** A real time PCR test for detection of RNA of dengue virus
- **Amplichain chikungunya:** A real time PCR test for detection of RNA of chikungunya virus
- **Amplichain HPV 16 and 18:** A real time PCR test for detection of DNA of HPV (16 and 18)
- **Amplichain HLA-B27:** A real time PCR test for detection of HLA-B27

Instrumentation

Amplichain Ex 32

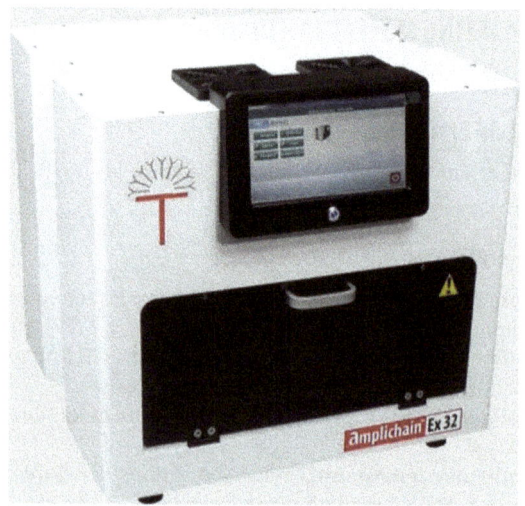

Fully automated nucleic acid extraction system.

Innovative Design

- ❖ Compatible with deep well plate for simultaneous processing of 16 × 2 samples.
- ❖ Individual test cartridge extraction system for simultaneous processing of 1 × 8 samples.

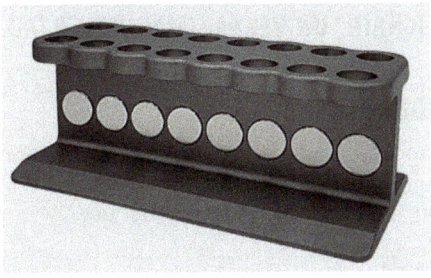

Magnetic Stand
Magnetic stand for manual nucleic acid extraction.

AMPLICHAIN® UNIVERSAL (MAGNETIC BEAD METHOD)

INTENDED USE

This kit is recommended to be used for the isolation of DNA/RNA from blood, serum, plasma and other body fluids using magnetic beads. This kit is for in vitro diagnostics use.

SUMMARY

AMPLICHAIN® Universal is a simple and efficient system for extraction and purification of total DNA/RNA from samples like blood, serum, plasma and other body fluids using magnetic beads and is utilized extensively for molecular biology research and is becoming an important tool in human clinical testing.

Principle

In the first step, the specimen is mixed with the lysis/binding buffer and magnetic beads during which the specimen is lysed and releases substantial amount of nucleic acids from the cells which bind to the magnetic beads. In the next step, the DNA/RNA bound to the beads are washed with wash buffer A and B substantially to remove the salts and proteins. Finally, the elution buffer is added to elute the DNA/RNA from the beads; eluted DNA/RNA can be used for PCR and other molecular testing.

Kit Components and Packaging Specifications

Each reagent kit contains reagents as follows. The expiry date of the unopened kit is stated on the outer label **(Table 5.1)**.

Table 5.1: Components of DNA/RNA extraction kit for PCR testing.

	Catalogue no.	Pack size	Presentation	Components and specifications
	1331020048	48T	Bulk pack	• Kit contains B1: Lysis/binding buffer. B2: magnetic beads B3: wash buffer A. B4: Qash buffer B. B5: elution buffer. For all open system instruments and manual usage
AMPLICHAIN® Universal	1332030016	16T	16 Prefilled individual test cartridges	• Prefilled individual cartridge containing lysis/binding buffer, magnetic beads, wash buffer A, wash buffer B and elution buffer • For AMPLICHAIN® Ex 32 or similar instruments
	1332010024	24T	24 Prefilled individual test cartridges	
	1332020096	96T	Prefilled test plate (16T × 6 plates)	• Prefilled plate containing lysis/binding buffer, magnetic beads, wash buffer A, wash buffer B and elution buffer • For AMPLICHAIN® Ex 32 or similar instruments

Storage and Stability of the Kit

(1) The kit and reagents are stored at 15–30°C. (2) Precipitate can be seen in the lysis/binding buffer when the buffer is stored at low temperature as it contains high concentration of salts. (3) Magnetic beads tend to settle with time. (4) It is necessary to mix the vials vigorously or vortex thoroughly so as to obtain a homogeneous mix.

Materials Required but Not Provided

(1) Magnetic Stand - MagStand^{TM} (1 No. - cat. no. 20221130060) and a microtube stand. (2) Nuclease inactivating agents such as DECON-R^{TM} (cat. no. 1108092000). (3) Incubator at 35°C (4) Dry bath up to 100°C (5) Nuclease free microtips (6) Micropipettes (7) Ethanol (96–100%) (8) RNase free water^{TM} (cat. no. 1108111250).

Warnings

- **AMPLICHAIN®** Universal lysis/binding buffer contains guanidine thiocyanate which is corrosive to metals, causes skin corrosion and serious eye damage.
- Recommended personal protective equipment includes dust mask type N95, eye shields and thick durable nitrile or plastic gloves.
- **If on skin:** Gently wash with plenty of water.
- If skin irritation or rash occurs get medical advice/attention. Kindly note that the lysis/binding buffer should not be used in a testing platform that uses bleach or in laboratories that use bleach as a part of their routine decontamination and disposal process. When the bleach interacts with guanidine thiocyanate, it produces the hazardous cyanide gas.

Precautions

- A thorough understanding of the pack insert is mandatory before performing the test for the first time. Adherence to protocol specified herein is necessary to ensure optimal performance of the product. Any deviation from the assay procedure may affect the results.
- Do not mix reagents of different lots.
- Do not use reagents beyond their expiry date.
- Use nuclease free plasticware and water.
- Avoid any contamination among samples; for this purpose, disposable tips should be used for each sample and reagent.
- Do not use reagents from other manufacturers along with the kit reagents for a given test run.
- Do not interchange reagent vials and their screw caps to avoid cross contamination. Use a clean, fresh, disposable pipette tip for each reagent or specimen manipulation.
- Always wear gloves. After wearing gloves, do not touch surfaces and equipment to avoid reintroduction of nuclease to material.
- Close reagent vials tightly immediately after use to avoid evaporation and microbial contamination.
- Treat surfaces of benches and glassware with commercially available nuclease inactivating agents.
- Use sterile, disposable nuclease-free plasticware.
- Use only DEPC-treated water or nuclease free water.
- Best results were obtained by using fresh samples or samples that have been quickly frozen in liquid nitrogen or stored at –70°C.
- Tubes and tips should be disposed into a waste bin containing 10% sodium hypochlorite solution to disinfect the consumables.
- Practice good laboratory practice (GLP) while handling specimens and other reagents.

Preparation of Reagents
*Only for Bulk Pack (Table 5.2)

Table 5.2: Reagents and its contents.

Reagents	Contents/labels	Volume of ethanol (96–100%) to be added
B1	Lysis/binding buffer	25 mL
B3	Wash buffer A	15 mL
B4	Wash buffer B	35 mL

Note: B1, B3 and B4 are supplied as concentrate. Before using for the first time, add recommended volume of ethanol (96–100%) as indicated above and on the respective bottles. Please tick mark the check box provided on the label after addition of ethanol.

Test Procedure
*Only for Bulk Pack

For Manual Method

- Bring the reagents and samples to room temperature before use.
- Pipette 800 µL of **B1 (lysis/binding buffer)** in a 2 mL microcentrifuge tube.
- Add 300–500 µL sample and mix well by pipetting up and down 10–15 times. (For quantitative test use 500 µL sample volume.)
- Place the tubes in heating block for 15 minutes at 70°C and for MTB samples at 90°C.
- After heating, add 15 µL of **B2 (magnetic beads)** and mix properly by pipetting up and down 10 to 15 times.
- Place the tubes in microtube stand and incubate for 15 minutes at RT.
- Following incubation, place the tube in a magnetic stand for 2 minutes. It will draw the magnetic bead/NA complex to the side

of the tube. Aspirate and discard the supernatant completely using a pipette without disturbing the magnetic bead/NA complex.
- Transfer the tubes to a normal microtube stand.
- Add 800 µL of **B3 (wash buffer A)** to the tube and thoroughly resuspend the beads by pipetting up and down 10–15 times.
- Place the tube in a magnetic stand for 2 minutes to draw the magnetic bead/NA complex to the side of the tube. Aspirate and discard the supernatant completely using a pipette without disturbing the mgnetic beads/NA complex.
- Transfer the tubes to a normal microtube stand.
- Add 800 µL of B4 (wash buffer B) to the tube and thoroughly resuspend the beads by pipetting up and down 10–15 times.
- Place the tube in a Magnetic stand for 2 minutes to draw the magnetic beads/NA complex to the side of the tube. Aspirate and discard the supernatant completely using a pipette without disturbing the magnetic bead/NA complex.
- Transfer the tubes to a normal microtube stand.
- Allow the magnetic bead/NA complex to air-dry by keeping the lids open for approx. 10 minutes, preferably in an incubator at 35°C. **Note:** It is important that the magnetic beads are dried completely before continuing with the elution step.
- Add 60 µL of **B5 (elution buffer)** to the tube and carefully resuspend the beads completely with microtip and by pipetting up and down 10 to 15 minutes.
- Incubate the suspension at 35°C for 10 minutes.
- Place the tube in a magnetic stand for 2 minutes to draw the magnetic beads to the side of the tube. Aspirate and collect the elute (~50 to 60 µL) completely using a pipette without disturbing the magnetic beads.
- Transfer the elute containing the purified DNA/RNA to a clean elute collection tube.

For AMPLICHAIN® Ex 32 or similar Nucleic Acid Extractors

- In a 96 deep well plate, add 500 µL of **B1 (lysis/binding buffer)** in the 1st and 7th well.
- In the 2nd and 8th well add 300 µL of ethanol and 20 µL of **B2 (magnetic beads)** and mix well.
- In the 3rd and 9th well, add 500 µL of **B3 (wash buffer A)**.
- In the 4th and 10th well add 500 µL of **B4 (wash buffer B)**.
- In the 6th and 12th well, add 120 µL of **B5 (elution buffer)**.
- Finally add 500 µL of test sample in the 1st and 7th well and place the plate in the **AMPLICHAIN® Ex 32**.
- Refer user manual of **AMPLICHAIN® Ex 32** or similar instruments for further instructions.
- The elutes are collected in a clean elute collection tube and tested by PCR run.

For Prefilled Individual Test Cartridge

AMPLICHAIN® Universal Individual test cartridge is prefilled with all reagent components. Refer user manual of **AMPLICHAIN® Ex 32** or similar instruments for further instructions.

For Prefilled Plate

AMPLICHAIN® Universal Plate is prefilled with all reagent components. Refer user manual of **AMPLICHAIN®** Ex 32 or similar instruments for further instructions.

Storage of Elute with Purified DNA/RNA

The elute contains pure DNA/RNA, recommended to be stored at lower temperature (-80°C). Avoid repeated freezing and thawing of the sample which may cause denaturing of DNA/RNA.

Assay Performance

Analytical specificity: The analytical specificity of **AMPLICHAIN® Universal** was evaluated by clinical testing of elutes of different cultures and different positive samples as listed below **(Table 5.3)**

Table 5.3: Analytical specificity using PCR.

Sr. no.	Organisms	Results
1	*Bacillus subtilis, Candida albicans, Enterococcus faecalis, Escherichia coli, Legionella, Pseudomonas aeruginosa, Salmonella enterica, Staphylococcus aureus, Staphylococcus epidermis, Streptococcus pyogenes, Mycobacterium tuberculosis* (MTB), Dengue virus, Chikungunya virus, HLA-B27, Hepatitis B virus, Hepatitis C virus, Human immunodeficiency virus	Positive amplification

Sample types analyzed: Culture extracts, blood, serum, plasma, sputum, and other body fluids.

Reproducibility and repeatability: AMPLICHAIN® Universal were used for extraction of MTB spiked samples on two different machines, by two users, and 3 different lots on 3 days to check the reproducibility and repeatability of the product. The extracted samples were tested using **AMPLICHAIN® MTB**. No discrepancy was observed implying the kits produces reproducible results and are consistent in its application.

The test was found to be reproducible with 100% detection rate and percent coefficient of variation <5% in terms of Ct values which is well below the accepted 10% across samples and between devices.

Clinical performance: The clinical performance of **AMPLICHAIN® Universal** was evaluated using clinical specimen in culture extracts, blood, serum, plasma, sputum, and other body fluids. A total of

150 specimens were extracted using **AMPLICHAIN® Universal** which were tested using **AMPLICHAIN®** PCR kits and HiPCR 16s rRNA SYBr PCR kit. Positive percent agreement (PPA) and negative percent agreement (NPA) were determined by comparing results of **AMPLICHAIN®** products relative to the results of the existing licensed kit **(Table 5.4)**

Table 5.4: Licensed Kit.

Extraction kit used	Positive samples	Negative samples
AMPLICHAIN® Universal	122	28
Existing licensed kit	122	28

Specificity: 100% Sensitivity: 100%

BIBLIOGRAPHY

1. Data on File, Tulip Diagnostics (P) Ltd., Molecular Diagnostics Division.
2. Pan S, Gu B, Wang H, Yan Z, Wang P, Pei H, et al. Comparison of four DNA extraction methods for detecting Mycobacterium tuberculosis by real-time PCR and its clinical application in pulmonary tuberculosis. J Thorac Dis. 2013;5(3):251-7.
3. Boom R, Sol CJA, Salimans MMM, Jansen CL, Wertheim-Van Dillen PME, Van Der Noordaa J. Rapid and sample method for purification of Nucleic Acids. The Netherlands Received 2 August 1989/Accepted 28 November 1989.
4. Witt S, Neumann J, Zierdt H, Gèbel G, Röscheisen C. Establishing a novel automated magnetic bead-based method for the extraction of DNA from a variety of forensic samples. Forensic Sci Int Genet. 2012;6(5):539-47.
5. Yang G, Erdman DE, Kodani M, Kools J, Bowen, MD, Fields BS. Comparison of commercial systems for extraction of nucleic acids from DNA/RNA respiratory pathogens. J. Virol. Methods. 2011;171(1):195-9.

SYMBOL KEYS

Temperature limitation	Consult instructions for use	Date of manufacture	**LOT** Batch number/lot number
Manufacturer	**IVD** In vitro diagnostic medical device	Contains sufficient for <n> tests	**REF** Catalogue number
Date of expiry	This side up	Caution	Corrosive

AMPLICHAIN CHIKUNGUNYA

(A real time PCR test kit for detection of RNA of Chikungunya Virus)

DESCRIPTION

The chikungunya virus (ChikV) is a single-stranded RNA virus that is transmitted to humans by the bite of the infected mosquitoes from the Aedes family. It is an RNA virus with a positive-sense single-stranded genome of about 11.6 kb and belongs to the alphavirus genus of the family Togaviridae. The symptoms typically include fever, headache, and a popular or maculopapular rash during the acute stage. Nucleic acid amplification-based assays or Real-time polymerase chain reaction (PCR) is a method that allows for sensitive and specific detection of chikungunya from clinical samples.

Intended Use

AMPLICHAIN® Chikungunya is a real-time PCR in vitro diagnostic test kit intended for the qualitative detection of chikungunya virus from the clinical samples like whole blood/serum/plasma in humans collected from individuals suspected of chikungunya infection by their healthcare provider. Positive results are indicative of presence of chikungunya virus RNA. The real-time PCR technique is considerably simple and fast with respect to the standard PCR technique. This technique has been successfully used for the rapid detection and identification of a variety of pathogens. AMPLICHAIN® Chikungunya is intended for use by qualified and trained clinical laboratory personnel specifically instructed and trained in the techniques of real-time PCR and in vitro diagnostic procedures.

Principle

AMPLICHAIN® Chikungunya uses TaqMan™-based real time PCR technique to conduct in vitro reverse transcription of chikungunya virus RNA, amplification of DNA and fluorescence detection. The assay targets specific genomic regions of nonstructural protein 2 (NSP2). This region is specific to chikungunya virus. The TaqMan™ probes for the target amplicons are labeled with FAM for target-specific signal. The assay includes housekeeping gene as internal control (IC) to monitor the processes from sample collection, nucleic acid extraction to fluorescence detection. The IC probe is labeled with HEX/VIC fluorescent dye to differentiate its fluorescent signal from chikungunya virus.

Kit Components and Packaging Specifications

Each reagent kit contains reagents for the pack sizes as mentioned in **Tables 5.5** and **5.6** below. Each of the reagents will be provided in separate zip-lock pouches. The expiry date of the unopened kit is stated on the outer label.

Table 5.5: Pack size mentioned number of test.

Catalogue no.	1313090016	1313090032	1323090048	1323090096
Pack size	16 Tests	32 Tests	48 Tests	96 Tests

Table 5.6: AMPLICHAIN® chikungunya kit component.

Component name	Pack size	Specifications	Main ingredients	Storage
R1: Master mix	16T	8 reactions × 2 PCR tube strips (lyophilized)	Taq DNA polymerase, MMLV, dNTPs, buffers, primers and probes	2–8°C
	32T	8 reactions × 4 PCR tube strips (lyophilized)		
	48T	24 reactions × 2 vials (lyophilized)		
	96T	24 reactions × 4 vials (lyophilized)		
R2: Reconstitution buffer	16T	250 µL × 1 Vial	Hot Start Buffer	2–8°C
	32T	250 µL × 2 Vials		
	48T	550 µL × 1 Vial		
	96T	550 µL × 2 Vials		
R3: Positive control	16T		Positive controls for chikungunya virus	2–8°C
	32T	8 reactions × 1 strip (lyophilized)		
	48T			
	96T	8 reactions × 2 strips (lyophilized)		
R4: No template control	250 µL × 1 Vial		Nuclease free water	2–8°C
RFID	Preprogrammed for AMPLICHAIN® qPCR instrument only			

Notes: (1) The reference materials and other components in the kit should be treated as potential sources of infection. (2) The use of this kit should be strictly in accordance with the nucleic acid amplification guidelines to operate in compliance with the requirements of the appropriate laboratories. (3) The components in different batches of the kit cannot be used interchangeably. (4) Do not use beyond expiration date.

Materials Required but Not Provided

(1) Biosafety cabinet (2) PCR hood (3) Calibrated variable micropipettes (capacity: 10 to 100 µL) (4) Sterile pipette filter tips (aerosol free) (maximum capacity 10 µL and 1,000 µL) (5) Any real time PCR machine compatible with FAM, CY5 and HEX/VIC dyes can be used with this kit. (6) PCR tubes—single/strips and caps (0.2/0.1 mL) or 96 well plate with optical sealer and PCR tube stand as recommended for the PCR instrument. (7) Cooling blocks (8) DECON-R^{TM} (cat. no. 1108092000) or similar for surface RNase decontamination (9) RNase free water^{TM} (Cat. no. 1108111250), AMPLICHAIN® nuclease free water (cat. no. 1351016500) (10) Sterile nitrile gloves (11) Facemask (N95) (12) Head cap (13) Lab coats/PPE kit (14) Negative extraction control (optional not provided) (15) Extraction kit (AMPLICHAIN® Universal) or any other manual or automated nucleic acid extraction methods can also be used.

Warnings and Precautions

(1) For in vitro diagnostic use only. (2) Positive results are indicative of the presence of target nucleic acid in the sample. (3) Keep the kit upright during storage and transportation. (4) Before using the kit, check vials for breakage, leakage, or damage. (5) All the liquid components of the kit should be thawed at room temperature and thoroughly mixed before use. (6) Read the procedure carefully before starting the experiment. (7) Wear protective gloves/protective clothing/eye protection/face protection. (8) Follow good clinical laboratory practices while handling clinical samples. Standard precautions should be followed as per established guidelines. Safety guidelines may be referred in safety data sheets of the product.

Steps to Avoid Cross-contamination

- Cross-contamination may occur when inappropriate handling of reference materials and specimens which will cause inaccurate results.
- Avoid microbial and nuclease (DNase/RNase) contamination of specimens and components of the kit. It is recommended to use sterile disposable filter-tips to aspirate reagents and specimens.
- All specimens to be tested and the reference materials of the kits should be considered as infectious substances and processed strictly in accordance with laboratory biosafety requirements.
- Sterile centrifuge tubes and filter-tips should be used.
- Store positive and/or potentially positive material separated from all other components of the kit.
- Take special precautions to avoid contamination of negative control.
- Do not open the reaction tubes/plates post amplification, to avoid contamination with amplicons.
- After use, the tips should be disposed into a waste bin containing a 2% sodium hypochlorite solution.
- After the operation, the work area surface and the instrument surface should be disinfected with a freshly prepared 2% sodium hypochlorite solution, and then cleaned with 70% ethanol or pure water. Finally, turn on UV light to disinfect working surfaces for 15 minutes.
- The PCR instrument used for this assay should be calibrated regularly according to instrument's instructions to eliminate cross-talks between channels. Discard sample and assay waste according to your local safety regulations.

Collection, Storage and Shipment of Specimens

- **Specimen type:** human whole blood, serum and plasma.
- **Sample preparation:** Samples need to be extracted and purified for high yield. For extraction and purification of viral nucleic acids we recommend using AMPLICHAIN® Universal as instructed in the protocol.
- **Storage and shipping:** Store specimens at 2–8°C for up to 48 hours after collection. Specimens must be packaged, shipped, and transported according to the current edition of dangerous goods regulation. Store specimens at 2–8°C and ship overnight to the lab on ice pack. Additional useful and detailed information on packing, shipping, and transporting specimens can be found at interim laboratory biosafety guidelines for handling and processing specimens.

PCR Working Area Requirements

This kit uses PCR-based technology, and experiments should be conducted ideally in three separate areas: specimen preparation area, reagent preparation area, amplification area. Personal protective equipment accessories (goggles, work clothes, hats, shoes, gloves, etc.) should be worn during operation and protective equipment accessories should be changed when entering and leaving different work areas. Protective equipment accessories in each work area are not interchangeable.

Storage and Handling of Amplichain® Chikungunya Reagents

(1) Store all reagents at 2–8°C after reconstitution. (2) If reagents get frozen, completely thaw the reagents at room temperature before use. (3) Use the reagents within 5 days once reconstituted.

Assay Procedure Nucleic Acid Extraction of the Specimens

(1) It should be performed in specimen preparation area. (2) Refer to extraction kit (**AMPLICHAIN® Universal**) package insert for detailed protocol. (3) Prepare specimens and place them in a biological safety cabinet. If the specimens are frozen, completely thaw them at room temperature and follow the nucleic acid extraction protocol. (4) All specimens should be handled as infectious, proper biosafety precautions including personal protective equipment must be used when handling specimen material.

Test Procedure

After nucleic acid extraction, setup PCR manually according to the procedures described below using AMPLICHAIN® Chikungunya in the dedicated reagent preparation area.

For 16 and 32 Test Pack Sizes

Reconstitution of lyophilized reagents:
- **To be performed only once for each kit before proceeding to PCR testing.**
- **R3: Positive control** is provided in lyophilized format in individual tubes. One tube is sufficient for one test/reaction.
- Detach the required number of positive control tubes and store the remaining tubes for further use.
- Reconstitute **R3: Positive control** with 10 µL of nuclease free water (NFW), give it a gentle swirl. Do not vortex.
- The kit contains **R1: Master mix** in PCR tubes. One PCR tube is sufficient for one test/reaction.
- The **R1: Master mix** is provided in lyophilized format to increase stability and maintain performance of the kit for longer duration.

- Detach the required number of PCR tubes from the strip and place it on the PCR rack. The remaining PCR tubes should be stored for further use.
- Thaw all the components thoroughly before using it. Mix gently by swirling the reconstituted vials and test it immediately.
- Remove the silicone stoppers from the PCR tubes and discard them aseptically.

In each of the PCR Tubes: R1: **Master mix, (Table 5.7)** add the following reagents as mentioned in the table below

Table 5.7: Master mix for 16 and 32 test pack sizes.

Component name	Specimen test Vol/test	Positive control (PC) Vol/test	No template control (NTC) Vol/test	NEC—human specimen negative extraction control Vol/test
R2: Reconstitution buffer	10 µL	10 µL	10 µL	10 µL
R3: Positive control	-	10 µL	-	-
R4: No template control	-	-	10 µL	-
NEC—human specimen negative extraction control	-	-	-	10 µL
Sample elute	10 µL	-	-	-
Total volume	20 µL	20 µL	20 µL	20 µL

For 48 and 96 Test Pack Sizes

Reconstitution of lyophilized reagents.

- **To be performed only once for each kit before proceeding to PCR testing.**
- The **R1: Master mix** is provided in lyophilized format to increase stability and maintain performance of the kit for longer duration.
- Reconstitute each vial of **R1: Master mix** with 250 µL of **R2: Reconstitution buffer** before use. Give it a gentle swirl. Do not vortex. It becomes a readymade single reagent format for daily testing. **(Table 5.8)**
- One vial of **R1: Master mix** is sufficient for 24 reactions. If the number of test samples is <24, only one vial can be reconstituted. The other vial can be reconstituted later whenever required.
- **R3: Positive control** is provided in lyophilized format in individual tubes. One tube is sufficient for one test/reaction.
- Detach the required number of positive control tubes and store the remaining tubes for further use.
- Reconstitute **R3: Positive control** with 10 µL of nuclease free water (NFW), give it a gentle swirl. Do not vortex.
- All reagents can be kept on cold racks during experimental set up.
- Thaw all the components thoroughly before using it. Mix gently by swirling the reconstituted vials and test it immediately.

Table 5.8: Master mix with 250 µL of R2: reconstitution buffer.

Component name	Reconstitution reagent	Volume of R2 to be added in R1	Storage
R1: Master mix	R2: Reconstitution buffer	250 µL	2–8°C or below

Experimental Setup (Table 5.9)

Table 5.9: Components of experimental setup.

Component name	Specimen test Vol/test	Positive control (PC) Vol/test	No template control (NTC) Vol/test	NEC—human specimen negative extraction control Vol/test
R1: Master mix	10 µL	10 µL	10 µL	10 µL
R3: Positive control	-	10 µL	-	-
R4: No template control	-	-	10 µL	-
NEC—Human specimen negative extraction control	-	-	-	10 µL
Sample elute	10 µL	-	-	-
Total volume	20 µL	20 µL	20 µL	20 µL

Test Controls

The following assay controls should be run concurrently with all test samples.

- ❖ PC - Positive control with an expected Ct value range (provided with the kit).
- ❖ NTC - No template control added during PCR reaction set-up (provided with the kit).
- ❖ NEC - Human specimen negative extraction control extracted concurrently with the test samples; provides extraction

procedural control and a secondary negative control that validates the extraction procedure and reagent integrity (not provided).

- Depending on total number of specimens, PC, NTC and NEC, dispense 10 µL into PCR tube or well of a 96-well PCR plate.
- Prior to moving to the specimen/nucleic acid handling area, prepare the no template control (NTC) reaction wells in the assay preparation area. Pipette 10 µL of R4: no template control into the NTC wells. Securely cap NTC wells before proceeding.
- Cover the entire reaction plate and move the reaction plate to the specimen/nucleic acid handling area.
- Add 10 µL of extracted nucleic acid into each designated tube or well containing PCR mix. Close lids of the PCR tubes or seal PCR plates with an appropriate film.
- Cover the entire reaction plate and move the reaction plate to the positive control handling area.
- Pipette 10 µL of **R3: Positive control** to the designated positive control well. Securely cap well.
- If necessary, briefly centrifuge them to get rid of bubbles.

Amplification

Note: Please ensure that the instruments have been installed, calibrated, checked, and maintained according to the manufacturer's recommendations.

For AMPLICHAIN® qPCR Instrument

RFID card provided in the kit contains preprogrammed parameters.
Please refer to the user manual of **AMPLICHAIN® qPCR.**

Other compatible real-time PCR instruments: Thermo Fisher, Qiagen and Bio-Rad. However, any real-time PCR instrument which uses FAM, HEX and CY5 dye can be used.

PCR Run Setup for Thermo Fisher Instruments

- Set up and run the real-time PCR instrument. Refer to real-time pcr instrument reference guide for detailed instructions.
- When setting up the targets and samples, create the following detectors with the quencher settings.
- The passive reference must be set as None.
- Sample volume to be set at 20 µL **(Table 5.10)**.

Table 5.10: Sample Volume to be set at 20 µL.

Target name or detector	Reporter	Quencher
Chikungunya **(NSP2)**	FAM	None
Internal control	HEX/VIC	None

PCR Run Setup for Rotor-Gene Q, QIAGEN Instruments (Table 5.11)

- Set up and run the real-time PCR instrument. Refer to the real-time PCR instrument reference guide for detailed instructions.

Table 5.11: PCR Run Setup for Rotor-Gene Q.

Target name or detector	Reporter/acquisition	Channel
Chikungunya (NSP2)	FAM	Green
Internal control	HEX/VIC	Yellow

- Perform optimization before first acquisition.
- Use positive control in the first position.

- ❖ For setting up the gains/gain optimization. Set gain method as: fixed. Define gain value as: 5. Do it for both channels green and yellow.
- ❖ Also check the temperature. It should be annealing temperature of our run method.
- ❖ The passive reference must be set as None.
- ❖ Sample volume to be set at 20 µL.

Sample Layout Details

- ❖ Set up the sample layout by assigning a unique sample name to each well.
- ❖ Assign a task to each well.
  - *Sample or Unknown:* For patient samples
  - *Standard or PC:* For positive control
  - *NTC:* For no template control
  - *NEC:* For negative extraction control

Run Method/Profile for PCR Amplification (Table 5.12)

Table 5.12: Temperature and time of amplification.

Step	Temperature	Time	Number of cycles
1	45°C	15 minutes	1
2	95°C	3 minutes	1
3	95°C	15 Seconds	45 cycles
4	55°C	25 Seconds*	

For 7500 ABI systems, 30 seconds to be selected.

- ❖ Collect fluorescence signal during the final 55°C step.
- ❖ Set the sample volume at 20 µL.
- ❖ Double check all settings then click Run or Start to initialize amplification.

Interpretation of Results

- **Baseline and threshold setting:** After the run completion, save and analyze the data according to the instrument instructions. Most instruments will automatically set up the background/baseline parameters and threshold level which will often produce acceptable results. In some cases, the background/baseline and threshold must be set manually for optimal results. The background/baseline usually starts from 3–5 cycles and ends a few cycles before any significant fluorescence amplification occurs. The threshold level should be set to the beginning of the exponential phase of amplification curves and above the background signal such as the signal from the no template control (NTC). Perform data analysis and interpret the results based on the tables listed in the sections "Quality Control" and "Examination and Interpretation of Specimen Results".

- **Quality control (Table 5.13):** Test results from positive control and no template control (NTC) should be examined prior to interpretation of specimen results. Positive control and no template control (NTC) should meet the requirements listed in the below table to ensure valid results. If the controls are not valid, the specimen results cannot be interpreted.

Table 5.13: Table of positive control and no template control (NTC) and negative extraction control.

Control	Ct values	
	Chikungunya (FAM)	Internal control (HEX/VIC)
No Template control (NTC)	Undetermined or (-ve) or >38*	Undetermined or (-ve) or >38*
Positive control (PC)	Ct ≤ 38	Ct ≤ 38
Negative extraction control (NEC)	Undetermined or (-ve)	Ct ≤ 38

*Refer to steps to avoid cross-contamination under WARNINGS AND PRECAUTIONS.

- **Examination and interpretation of specimen results (Table 5.14)**: Assessment of clinical specimen test results should be performed after the positive and negative controls have been examined and confirmed to be valid and acceptable. If the controls are not valid, the patient results cannot be interpreted. The table below lists the expected results for the kit with valid positive control and negative control. Ct cut-off targets presented below are derived from product verification and validation studies, and user should determine own Ct cut-off values for optimal performance.

Table 5.14: Examination and interpretation of specimen results.

Ct		
Internal control (HEX/VIC)	**Chikungunya (FAM)**	*Result interpretation*
Ct ≤ 38	Undetermined or (-ve)	Chikungunya not detected
No requirements on the Ct value	Ct ≤ 38	Chikungunya detected
Ct ≤ 38	Ct ≥ 38	Re-extraction and re-test recommended
Undetermined or (-ve)	Undetermined or (-ve)	Invalid result, specimen needs to be re-tested from re-extraction or recollected from patient for re-test

Limitations of the Procedure

(1) This kit is used for qualitative detection of chikungunya RNA from human whole blood/serum/plasma samples. The results cannot directly reflect the viral load in the original specimens. (2) This kit is only applicable to specimen types described in the section "INTENDED USE". Testing other types of specimens may

cause inaccurate results. The specimens to be tested shall be collected, processed, stored and transported in accordance with the conditions specified in the instructions. Inappropriate specimen preparation and operation may lead to inaccurate results. (3) The specimens to be tested shall be collected, processed, stored and transported in accordance with the conditions specified in the instructions. Inappropriate specimen preparation and operation may lead to inaccurate results. (4) Extraction and amplification of nucleic acid from clinical samples must be performed according to the specified methods listed in this procedure. Other extraction approaches and processing systems must be evaluated before use. (5) Primers and probes for this kit target highly conserved regions within the genome of chikungunya virus. (6) Negative results do not preclude chikungunya infection and should not be used as the sole basis of patient treatment/management decision. All results should be interpreted by a trained professional considering and reviewing the patient's medical history and clinical signs and symptoms.

Disposal Methods

Users must ensure safe disposal by autoclaving or incinerating the components after the test procedure. Please follow the recommended biohazard disposal and safety guidelines.

ASSAY PERFORMANCE

Analytical Specificity/Cross Reactivity (Table 5.15)

The analytical specificity of AMPLICHAIN® Chikungunya was evaluated by in silico testing and clinical testing. In silico analysis **(Table 5.16)** was performed by performing BLAST analysis of sequences of different commonly found bacteria and fungi (obtained from NCBI database) to show that the genetic sequences used in the primers and probes of the targets are not homologous.

Clinical evaluation of analytical specificity was performed by testing elutes of different cultures obtained after extraction with AMPLICHAIN® Chikungunya Master mix. Chikungunya samples were also tested. The list of samples tested in silico and clinically are listed as follows:

Table 5.15: Cross reactivity using PCR.

Organisms	Results
Bacillus subtilis, Candida albicans, Enterococcus faecalis, Escherichia coli, Legionella, Pseudomonas aeruginosa, Salmonella enterica, Staphylococcus aureus, Staphylococcus epidermis, Streptococcus pyogenes, Cytomegalovirus, Hepatitis B virus, Hepatitis C virus, Human Immunodeficiency Virus, Human papilloma virus	No amplification

Table 5.16: In silico evaluation using NCBI nucleotide BLAST.

Organisms	Chikungunya Forward/reverse primers, probe
Acinetobacter anitratus, Bacillus subtilis, Candida albicans, Enterobacter cloacae, Enterococcus faecalis, Escherichia coli, Gardnerella vaginalis, Legionella, Pseudomonas aeruginosa, Salmonella enterica, Staphylococcus aureus, Staphylococcus epidermis, Streptococcus mutans, Streptococcus pyogenes, Trichomonas vaginalis, Adenovirus, Cytomegalovirus, Epstein-Barr virus, Hepatitis B virus, Hepatitis C virus, Herpes simplex virus, Human immunodeficiency virus, Human papilloma virus, Simian virus	No similarity

Analytical Sensitivity (Limit of Detection)

The analytical sensitivity (Limit of detection) of AMPLICHAIN® Chikungunya was evaluated by testing with serial dilutions of chikungunya positive control (plasmid) prepared with nuclease free water. The concentration of the dilutions is in copies/mL. The limit of detection for chikungunya is 201.42 copies/mL.

Reproducibility and Repeatability

AMPLICHAIN® Chikungunya kit was tested for reproducibility and repeatability in 2 different PCR machines by 2 operators with 3 different lots of AMPLICHAIN® Chikungunya kits for 3 days with 10 samples. No discrepancies were observed in the testing. The test was found to be reproducible with a percent coefficient of variation <5% which is well below the acceptance criteria of 10% across samples and between devices. Refer to data on file, Tulip Diagnostics (P) Ltd., Molecular Diagnostics Division.

Clinical Performance (Table 5.17)

- ❖ **Internal evaluation:** The clinical performance of AMPLICHAIN® Chikungunya was evaluated using clinical specimens in whole blood/serum/plasma. A total of 82 specimens were tested using AMPLICHAIN® Chikungunya along with an existing licensed kit. Positive percent agreement (PPA) and negative percent agreement (NPA) were determined by comparing results of AMPLICHAIN® Chikungunya relative to the results of the existing licensed Kit.
- ❖ **External evaluation:** A total of 100 random samples were taken which includes samples from patients suspected for chikungunya infection. A total of 100 comparative runs with

three different manufacturing lots were performed to access the specificity and sensitivity of "AMPLICHAIN® Chikungunya".

Table 5.17: Clinical performance.

Kits used	Internal evaluation			External evaluation		
	Positive samples	Negative samples	Total	Positive samples	Negative samples	Total
AMPLICHAIN® Chikungunya	63	19	82	21	79	100
Existing licensed kit	63	19	82	21	79	100

- **Specificity:** 19 negative runs in internal evaluation and 79 negative runs in external evaluation correlated between the methods, depicting 100% specificity for AMPLICHAIN® Chikungunya.
- **Sensitivity:** 63 positive sample runs in internal evaluation and 21 positive sample runs in external evaluation correlated between the methods, depicting 100% sensitivity for AMPLICHAIN® Chikungunya.

In Use Stability Study

AMPLICHAIN® Chikungunya kit was tested for in use study to show the degree of stability of the product at 2–8°C under open vial influencing factor. Study was conducted over a period of 6 days. It was shown that the product remains stable for 6 days and after the 6th day, it starts deteriorating.

BIBLIOGRAPHY

1. Chikungunya fact sheet—WHO | World Health Organization https://www.who.int
2. Data on File, Tulip Diagnostics (P) Ltd., Molecular Diagnostics Division.
3. James Versalovic, Karen C. Carroll, Guido Funke, James H. Jorgensen, Marie Louise Landry, David W. Warnock (ed). Manual of Clinical Microbiology. 10th Edition. ASM Press, 2011.
4. Kularatne SAM. et al. Concurrent outbreaks of Chikungunya and Chikungunya fever in Kandy, Sri Lanka, 2006-07: a comparative analysis of clinical and laboratory features. Postgrad Med J. 2009;85:342-46.
5. Mishra N, James Ng, Jennifer L Rakeman, Michael J Perry, Dominick A Centurioni, Amy B Dean, et al. One-step pentaplex real-time polymerase chain reaction assay for detection of zika, dengue, chikungunya, West nile viruses and a human housekeeping gene, J. Clin. Virol. Volume 120.

ANY PARAMETER PCR TESTING FOLLOWS THE SAME PROCEDURAL PROTOCOLS BARRING A FEW REAGENT CHANGES

AVAILABLE PARAMETERS COMMERCIALLY WORLD OVER

MTB	Test for *Mycobacterium tuberculosis*
MTB-RIF	Test for Rifampicin Resistant *Mycobacterium tuberculosis*
MTB-INH	test for Isoniazid Resistant *Mycobacterium tuberculosis*
HAV	Test for hepatitis A virus
HBV	Test for hepatitis B virus
HCV	Test for hepatitis C virus
HEV	Test for hepatitis E virus
HIV-1	Test for HIV-1 virus
HIV-1/HIV-2	Test for HIV-1/HIV-2 virus
H1N1	Test for H1N1
H3N2/H1N1	Test for H3N2 and H1N1
CT	Test for *Chlamydia trachomatis*
NG	Test for *Neisseria gonorrhoeae*
CT/NG	Test for *Chlamydia trachomatis* and *Neisseria gonorrhoeae*
Trich	Test for *Trichomonas vaginalis*
Dengue	Test for dengue
Chikungunya	Test for chikungunya
Dengue/Chikungunya	Test for dengue and chikungunya
Malaria Pf	Test for *Plasmodium falciparum*
Malaria Pv/Pf	Test for *Plasmodium vivax* and *Plasmodium falciparum*

Salmonella	
LTS	Test for Leptospira
Shigella	Test for Shigella spp.
Scrub T	Test for Scrub typhus
Rabies	Test for rabies virus
HLA-B27	Test for HLA-B27
HPV-HR	Test for Human Papillomavirus high risk types 16, 31 and 18, 45
Nipah	Test for Nipah virus
GBS	Group B streptococcus
Influenza A/B	Test for influenza A and influenza B virus
Beta CoV	Test for beta coronavirus
COVID-19	Test for COVID-19
SARS CoV-2	Test for COVID-19
CDI	Test for *Clostridium difficile*
HSV (1/2)	Test for herpes simplex virus 1 and herpes simplex virus 2
Cholera	Test for cholera
HPV-HR 16 & 18	Test for human papillomavirus high risks types 16 and 18
HPV-HR 16, 18/31, 39, 45	Test for human papillomavirus high risks types 16, 18/31, 39, 45
Staph/MRSA	Test for *Staphylococcus aureus* and methicillin resistant *Staphylococcus aureus*
ZIKA	Test for Zika virus
MTB-FQ	Test for Fluoroquinolone resistant *Mycobacterium tuberculosis*
MTB/NTM	Test for *Mycobacterium tuberculosis* and nontuberculous mycobacteria
CMV	Test for *Cytomegalovirus*

Mumps	Test for mumps virus
Dengue/zika	Test for dengue and zika virus
Rubella/measles	Test for rubella and measles virus
Staph/PA	Test for *Staphylococcus aureus* and *Pseudomonas aeruginosa*
Inf A, B/COVID-19	Test for Influenza A, B and COVID-19
Rota V	Test for rotavirus
Mucormycosis	Test for mucormycosis
M. leprae	Test for *Mycobacterium leprae*
MPX	Test for monkeypox virus
Leish	Test for leishmaniasis
Mgen	Test for *Mycoplasma genitalium*
MTB COVID-19	Test for *Mycobacterium tuberculosis* and COVID-19
Syphilis	Test for *Treponema pallidum*
PA	Test for *Pseudomonas aeruginosa*
S. pneumoniae	Test for *Streptococcus pneumoniae*
Truenat® KFDV	Test for Kyasanur forest disease
Truenat® HIB	Test for *Haemophilus influenzae* type B
Truenat® Nm	Test for *Neisseria meningitides*
JEV	Test for Japanese encephalitis virus
RSV	Test for respiratory syncytial Virus (RSV)
SCD	Test for sickle cell disease

CHAPTER 6

Histopathology (Prelude to Immunohistochemistry)

INTRODUCTION

This book comprises of molecular pathology technology, techniques, and protocols mainly PCRS and immunohistochemistry. Imunohistochemistry comprises of technical preparation guide for specimen removed out of body during surgery, aspirates, body fluids. Macroscopic and microscopic examination (*Histopathology-by Greek definition histos–tissue; pathos–suffering; logia–study of*) of the specimen enables understanding of changes occurred in the disease and diagnose, on basis of which the medical treatment starts. Tissue has to undergo various stages of processing for preparation to a microscopic slide for evaluation (*histotechnology*). This involves tissue processing, embedding, microtomy, staining and mounting.

Histotechnician/histotechnologist are trained personnel with excellent mechanical skills, having expertise on equipments and knowledge of anatomy, science of tissue processing and various chemical reaction in staining protocol. They play a very important role in preparation of slide for microscopic evaluation. Preparation of slides for frozen sections, routine H&E stain, special stains like PAS, rectic, masson and many more, Immunohistochemistry. Molecular tests have become important ancillary tests identifying type of tumors for diagnosis, prognosis, and therapeutic aspect.

The sensitivity of the technique has improved over a period of years from immunofluorescence labeled antibody system to labeled polymer-based systems and also overcome the effects of formalin fixation for identifying epitopes. With the introduction of digital pathology, it is essential to monitor quality of slide preparation.

Understanding Basics of Tissue Processing (Fig. 6.1)

Action for removal of water.

Water is found in tissue in two forms, free and bound water. The bound water molecule is an integral part of macromolecules of the cell. Proteins, lipids, carbohydrates, and nucleic acids are major macromolecules of the cell having their own specific function within living cells. Correct dehydration defines removal of free water, leaving bound water intact.

- ❖ **Fixation and gross examination:** Fixation is the process of preserving tissue from decomposing and are placed in a solution called fixative. All fixative solutions are aqueous in nature.
- ❖ Gross examination is the macroscopic observation and dissection of tissue for purpose of diagnosis.

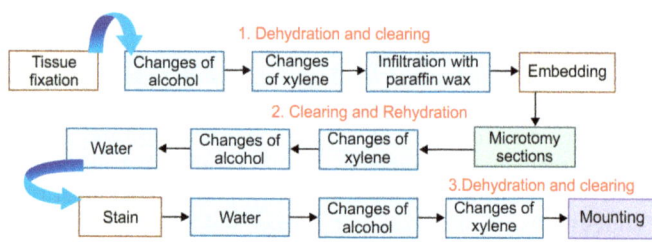

Fig. 6.1: Basics of tissue processing cycle—dehydration-rehydration-dehydration.

- ❖ **Processing and embedding—step 1:** Paraffin wax is universally used for embedding tissue section. Most of the fixatives used for tissue preservation are aqueous solutions. Water is removed from aqueous fixed tissue sections using changes of alcohol and alcohol is removed using xylene making place for paraffin wax to infiltrate. This process hardens tissue and helps in section cutting.
- ❖ **Microtomy:** Microtomy is an art by means of which tissue is cut into thin sections. A microtome is an instrument used for cutting sections.
- ❖ **Staining and mounting—step 2:** Staining procedure imparts color to tissue components which can be visualized under microscope. Paraffin wax is removed using xylene and sections are brought to water treating with alcohol.
- ❖ **Mounting:** After staining is complete tissue sections dehydrated, cleared, and are mounted using mounting medium DPX—**step 3**.

TISSUE FIXATION AND GROSS EXAMINATION

Histopathology Specimen

Specimens received for histopathology examination are mainly collected by surgeons in the operation theatre. They are removed out of the body using various techniques at the time of surgery.

Specimens are received for examination in form of:
- ❖ **Incision biopsy:** Only portion of the lesion is sampled from suspected area usually sent for confirmation by frozen section.
- ❖ **Excision biopsy:** The entire lesion is removed usually with the rim of normal tissue. Therefore, this serves both diagnostic and therapeutic purpose.

- **Punch biopsy:** Small round tissue is removed using punch of desired diameter. Useful in lesions from skin, vulva, cervix.
- **Cone biopsy:** Cone shaped piece of lesion is removed from cervix.
- **Wedge biopsy:** Triangle shaped tissue lesion with small amount of normal tissue around it
- Biopsies are collected using Tru-cut needle, endoscope, CT/MRI, trephine needle.
- **Surgical resection:** Lumpectomy specimens, uterus, lymph nodes, gallbladder, Appendix
- **Complete resection:** Breast, kidney, intestine, larynx
- Amputations/limbs
- Slides and blocks for second opinion or ancillary tests

Accessioning of Specimen

Every specimen must be submitted with a complete requisition form **(Fig. 6.2)**.

Requisition must include:
- **Patient demographic details:** Name/Age/Sex
- OPD/IPD No./Bed. No./Ward
- Specimen site/Nature of operation
- Clinical notes by clinician/surgeon
- **Details of investigations:** Blood reports, CT/MRI/USG findings, X-rays
- Information of previous surgery, biopsy, cytology, PAP smear reports for correlation and documentation
- **Nature of specimen sent:** Tissue/slides/paraffin blocks/smears
- Details of tests billed

Histopathology requisition form

Patient name: Date:/___/

Age:_____ Years_____Sex:_____ Histopathology previous
Bed no: _____/Ward:- _____OPD/IPD no. no.

To be filled by the doctor

Nature of operation/procedure done:

Material sent:

Brief history:

Relevant past history:

Previous surgeries:

Investigations:

Treatment resolved [phase a tick]:

Chemotherapy   Radiotheraphy   Any other

To be filled by the i ar only

Nature of material received:
Second option: Number of blocks:_____Number of sliders/smears___-
Blocks/ slides/smears no:-_____

Forum-section	Small specimen	Medium specimen	Large specimen	Large R complex	FNAC	PAP smears	IHC	FISH/PCR

Fig. 6.2: Requisition form.

Specimen Identification and Receiving

This step involves receiving of specimen in the department for processing and reporting.

Specimens are received in the department from OT or OPD in the hospital and are also received in standalone/corporate laboratories by walk ins and nursing homes.

On receiving specimen in the department verify patient identification and information on the requisition form and the specimen container is matching with each other along with the tally of number of containers received. Also, observe and document the condition in which the specimen is received, fresh and unfixed, fixed inadequate or adequate formalin or autolyzed.

Labeling of Specimens

This is very important that specimens are properly accessioned and signed with a specific identification number as soon as specimen is received. This number should remain throughout entire processing steps and then in record keeping. This number includes organization identity/serial number/year – ABC/123/22. This number can be defined manually or also can be generated from software. Labeling should be done very carefully. Printed labels will take care of errors of manual labeling. Use lead pencil to label cassettes and slides as this number will remain during processing and staining. Also, use of Tissue Tek/Vogel system can be done which allows labeling of cassettes and slides. These numbers are retained permanently during processing and storage. Laboratory information system (LIS), automated labeling system will increase efficiency of laboratory by reducing labeling errors. Barcode labels are scanned for confirming identity at every step.

Fig. 6.3: Bar code.

Maintain a logbook for specimens received in the department. This register will include: Date received, Department serial number, Patient ID (in case of Hospital patient), Patient demography, Referring Doctor, Specimen details, and Diagnosis.

Histopathology Register

Date	HP no.	Patient ID	Patient name	Age/sex	Ref. by	Specimen	Diagnosis

Criteria for Specimen Rejection

As per NABL112 criteria *histopathology specimens should not be rejected on the ground of poor specimen integrity.*

- Specimen with no label/incorrect label:
  - Lack of minimum information on requisition
  - Specimen site
  - Date and time of collection
  - Patient's demographic data
  - Referring doctor's name
- Container label if does not match with requisition form
- **Incomplete requisition form:** Missing information of/incorrect specimen site details, patient's demographic details
- Improperly packed specimen/fixative leaked on requisition form
- **Specimen improperly fixed:** On receipt of specimen change fixative; add appropriate quantity of fixative into specimen bottle; document the same on the requisition form.
- **Slides broken beyond repair on receipt:** Inform to the source from where the sample is received; ask for the repeat sample if possible; document in the specimen discrepancy log.
- **Lost specimens:** Rare occasion but needs to be documented in criteria for rejection.

Rejected specimens are to be kept on hold and all possible efforts must be made to get the correct information from source as per NABL criteria.

Details including reason for rejection is entered in a specially maintained rejection logbook.

Gross Examination of Specimen

Gross examination is visual observation/description of specimen/dissection for submitting representative sections for processing. Primary responsibility of grossing is of pathologist. Histotechnician is responsible for fixation of specimens, arranging specimens, assisting pathologist during grossing and processing of tissue. Hence, it is important to understand grossing protocol.

Grossing Room

- **Safe grossing:** Use apparel (protective gear and clothing) which includes apron, closed shoes, mask, safety goggles and good quality snugly fitting gloves.
- Grossing room needs to be well equipped with proper ventilation, exhaust fan, proprietary grossing station, grossing board, weigh balance.
- **Grossing instruments (Figs. 6.3 and 6.4):**
- Straight and curved scissors (small and large, with pointed and blunt ends)
- Scalpel blades with handles
- Forceps (fine and toothed)
- Metal probe, saw
- A ruler
- Paint brush, ink and stainless-steel bowls of varying sizes
- Knives of various lengths

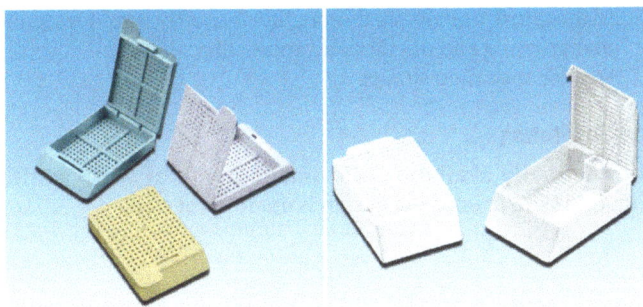

Fig. 6.3: Cassettes for tissue processing.

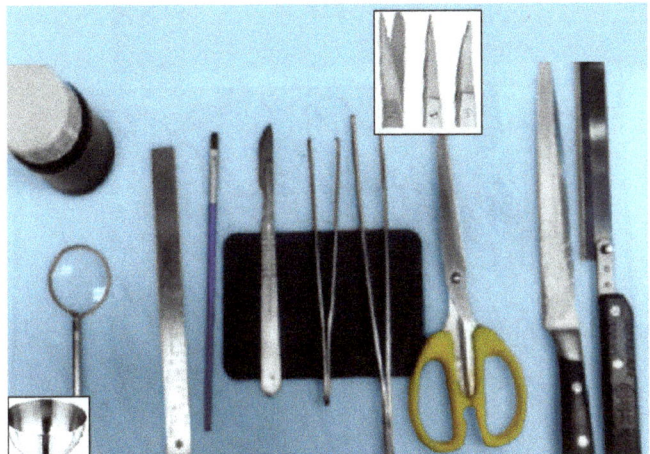

Fig. 6.4: Grossing cutting tools.

❖ All these instruments are thoroughly cleaned before, during and after grossing and dried to prevent rusting.
❖ Area for specimen storage

Grossing Station

Commercially available tailor-made modular work station **(Fig. 6.5)** with ergonomic design is made up of steel.

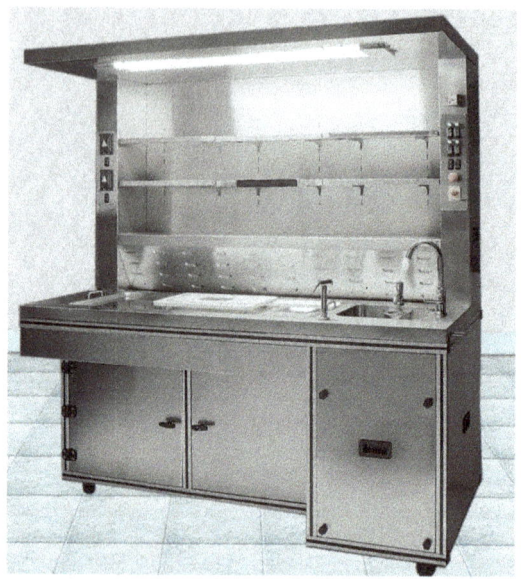

Fig. 6.5: Work station.

Salient Features

- Cutting board
- Rinsing facility on work surface
- While working removal of accumulated formalin and tissue waste below perforated sheet through fully programmed spray system.
- Waste grinder to avoid blockage of drainage system.
- Emergency pullout eye washer
- Backdraft extraction of formalin fumes with maximum efficiency
- Air filtration system to minimize hazardous fumes in the laboratory.

Method

- Arrange all specimens according to the prescriptions. The specimen along with the requisitions are once again to be verified before the grossing begins.
- Open the container of specimen in serial order with gloves in hand.
- Take out specimen, and observe for the gross appearance.
- Take the dimensions with a measuring scale. (a) Weight (b) Size (length, breadth, width) (c) Shape (d) Color (e) Visible abnormality (f) Internal abnormality (if present try to detect by an appropriate cut). Bits are submitted from both pathological and normal looking areas.
- Write the gross description on the receipt.
- Small specimens are fixed after noting all the gross features namely size, shape, color, consistency, hemorrhage, necrosis, etc. In small specimens, inking is of help during embedding.
- Cut specimens and take small sections from representative area. Put smaller bits in appropriately labelled jar containing fixative.

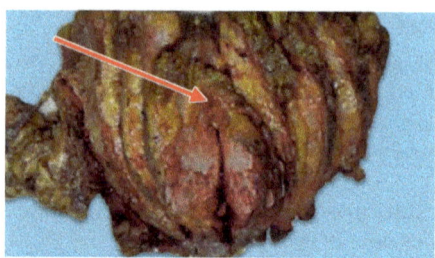

Fig. 6.6: Breast tumor cut in slices for better fixation.

- In the case of biopsy or small specimens submit whole specimen for processing.
- Big resection specimens are preliminarily examined for salient features and the external surface is painted with marking ink. The specimen is then cut opened or bisected or sliced (**Fig. 6.6**) in a regular manner taking care to avoid distortion and facilitate formalin penetration by keeping for overnight fixation. These specimens are grossed the next day by pathologist (**Fig. 6.7**).
- After grossing tissues are filled in cassettes along with appropriate identification number for further processing.
- Tiny tissue bits are wrapped in filter paper and eosin is added if too tiny to recognize during cutting.
- Entry of tissue bits selected for each specimen are entered in the gross entry book.
- Bony specimens are cut using band saw and are subjected for decalcification.
- Digital images whole specimen is captured before inking and dissecting specimen and also cut surface to demonstrate lesion.

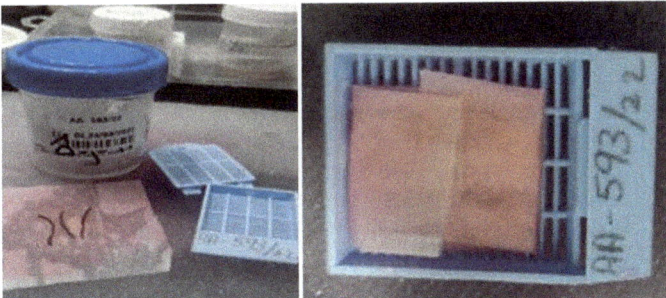

Fig. 6.7: Handling core biopsy.

The date of grossing and the name of the pathologist performing grossing is entered in the requisition. Also, document who's picking sections and number of cassettes.

A key for specimen is summary of noting number of cassettes/blocks for the specimen for, e.g., margins of resection, deepest penetration of tumor, tumor proper breast quadrants, lymph node levels.

The gross description of the specimens is written in detail. Ancillary techniques if identified must be noted, e.g., fungus stain or stains for kidney biopsy, liver biopsy, bone marrow.

Tissue loading work sheet

Date:						
Sr. no.	Specimen ID	Key for specimen blocks	Total no. of blocks	More sections	Sign	Remarks

Orientation of Specimen

- **Small specimens:** Endoscopic biopsies are submitted by placing the base of the biopsy on card paper.
- For wide excision specimens margins can be identified with sutures of different length and color. Specimens like breast lumpectomies and wide excisions can be oriented by means of sutures, ink, or clips. Specimens also signify orientation with their anatomical structure; For, e.g., axillary tail in mastectomy specimen **(Figs. 6.8A and B)**.
- Specimens received with staples and suture are neatly resected with scissors as close to the staple line as possible and subsequently the tissue next to it is submitted as margin taking care that the submitted tissue is free of staples or sutures.
- Stents and guide wire are not handled with gloves but are removed with toothed forceps as they have sharp ends.

Gross description involves,
- Type of surgical procedure for, e.g., uterus with bilateral adnexa, radical mastectomy

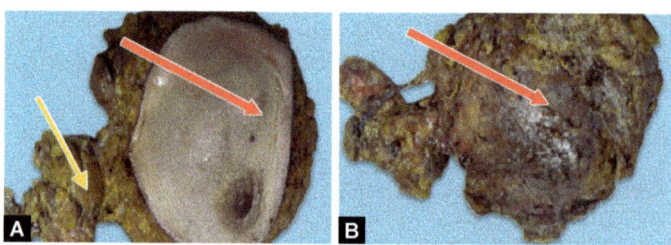

Figs. 6.8A and B: Breast tissue with axillary tail (Yellow arrow) + Tumor (Red arrow).

- ❖ **Anatomic site:** Appendix, gallbladder
- ❖ **Specimen type:** Tru-cut needle biopsy whether the specimen is received fresh or is immersed in formalin
- ❖ **Dimensions:** Length, breadth, and width + weight of the specimen are recorded before dissection. TUR prostate chips, solid organs such as uterus, spleen, kidneys etc., are weighed.
- ❖ **Specimen description:** Shape, color, surface appearance (external/internal)
- ❖ **Anatomic component description in case of resection:** On opening site and size of the tumor, location, distance from resection margins, presence of lymph nodes, vascular invasion is documented.

Tissue Fixation

Tissue fixation is an initial but critical step in preservation of morphological features of cells during the entire processing. Effects of tissue fixation/tissue processing can be appraised only when observed under microscope. Use of fixatives and duration of fixation vary widely between laboratories. Standardization of tissue fixation protocol is need of hour at the advent of several technological evolutions from H&E stain—special stains—immunohistochemistry (IHC) – FISH – PCR – next generation sequencing, i.e., testing and analyzing multiple genes on formalin fixed paraffin embedded tissue blocks (FFPE). Optimization of tissue fixation time, ratio of fixative to tissue and fixation criteria for specimen types from small biopsy to resections is very important steps in the fixation process.

Formaldehyde is universally used as fixative in form of aqueous solution for over a century now where, commonly used formulations of formaldehyde are 10% formal saline [neutral buffered formalin (NBF)].

Effects of Incomplete or Poor Tissue Fixation

Tissue processing	Poor quality sections; tissue gets lifted from slide unevenly or float completely. Cannot withstand retrieval techniques
Staining H&E	Nuclei smudging, bubbling, loss of nuclear chromatin or no nuclei staining, cell shrinkage and more eosinophilia in H&E stain
Immunohistochemistry	Loss of antigenicity resulting in no staining, nonspecific staining due to diffusion of antigens, tissue lifting, wrinkles, folds of tissue section and variable staining
ISH/FISH	Tissue loss complete or partial, loss of signals, impaired RNA/DNA extraction; enzyme digestion standardization fails

The best results of tissue preservation are obtained by putting tissue into fixative as soon as possible after surgery. *As per CAP guidelines, cold ischemic time is defined as time from excision of tissue during surgery to initiation of tissue fixation. Guidelines recommend interval time of ≤ one hour. However, tissue must be placed in fixative immediately after removed out of body by surgical procedure.*

The common causes of poor cellular details in histological preparation are autolysis and putrefaction.

Autolysis is the destruction of cells or tissues by enzymes liberated as a result of rupture of the lysozyme. The lytic enzymes are cathepsins, some of which are proteinases. These enzymes continue their metabolic processes even after interruption of blood supply until something happens to stop the enzyme action.

Putrefaction means breaking down of tissue by bacterial action often with the formation of gas resulting in decomposition.

Fixation is the process which preserves cells and tissue components close to living from acts by minimizing the loss of enzymatic destruction of cellular and extracellular molecules by maintaining macromolecular structure and protecting the tissues from destruction by bacterial action. This also protects tissues during all subsequent events such as processing steps, i.e., dehydration, embedding, sectioning followed by different staining protocols.

Definition

Fixation is defined as process in which cells or tissue are fixed in physical state and partly chemical state so that they will withstand subsequent treatment with various reagents with minimal loss distortion or decomposition.

Fixative

As soon as cells or tissues removed out of body it starts decomposing if left at room temperature. Hence tissue is immediately placed into fixative as soon as possible. Fixative preserves cells and tissue components for preparation of tissue for microscopy.

It plays important role in,
- Preserving tissue from autolysis and putrefaction
- Penetrate the tissue evenly with rapid action.
- Hardening of tissue during subsequent processing steps
- Conversion of semi fluid consistency of cells to an irreversible semisolid consistency.
- Alteration of refractive indices to varying degrees, which increases visibility or contrast of unstained components to be seen more easily.

10% of formaldehyde with the pH adjusted to physiological range 7.2–7.4 is commonly used worldwide as fixative.

Factors Affecting Fixation Process

- ❖ **Duration + penetration capacity:** Tissue fixation time and penetration capacity varies depending on tissue type. For achieving it is important that fixative penetrates form the periphery of the tissue to the center of tissue hence thickness of tissue section bit should be <4 mm **(Fig. 6.9)**. Endoscopic biopsies, Tru-cut needle biopsies can be fixed faster as compared to resected specimens.
- ❖ The type of fixative used, duration of fixation has important role in demonstration of antigen antibody and also in DNA/RNA extraction.

  Adequate duration for tissue fixation—6 to 24 hours

  For routine processing schedule thickness of tissue should be 2–4 mm thick.

  - Resected specimens, e.g., uterus, intestine etc., are cut open, spleen, breast, kidney or any organ, large tumor are sliced and fixed so that fixative can reach in contact with all surfaces of specimen. Also cotton or cloth soaked in the

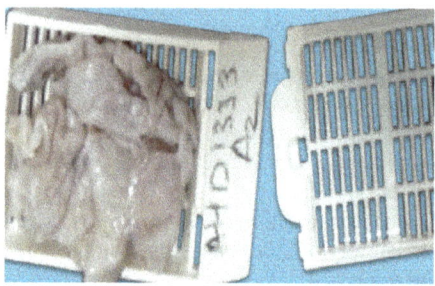

Fig. 6.9: Over sized chunks of tissue—incorrect way of loading tissue for processing.

fixative place at bottom of container will allow better outer surface fixation.
- Tissue must be left for an adequate time in fixative to avoid distortion during subsequent processing steps.
- Agitation improves penetration resulting in better infiltration and impregnation of the tissue.

❖ **Use of adequate fixative:** The quantity of fixative required for fixing specimen is 15–20 times that of the size of tissue (*See* **Fig. 6.10**). The container for the specimen should be appropriate to size of tissue. As per definition, the action of tissue fixation is chemical dependent. The process involves interaction of tissue constituents and chemical composition of fixative. If fixative volume is not in proportion tissue constituents will alter chemical composition of fixative resulting in poor fixation. Appropriate volume ratio of fixative with tissue will allow increase in penetration rate by covering all surfaces of tissue.

❖ **Temperature:** Increase in temperature will accelerate the fixation process. Tissue of 3–4 mm thickness can be fixed for 1–2 hours at 55 to 60°C, however routinely tissues are submitted for fixation at room temperature. For electron microscopy the range is chosen is 0–4°C.

❖ **pH, buffers:** pH of fixative is adjusted to physiological range, 7.2–7.4 using buffer solution. Unbuffered solution of formalin become acidic by reacting with atmospheric oxygen forming formic acid. 10% formal saline with the addition of sodium chloride also achieves correct osmolality, but the same can become acidic on long standing. This results in formation of formalin pigment (birefringent crystal) in the tissue section and variation in staining such as nuclear fading.

❖ **Concentration (Fig. 6.10):** 10% concentration of formalin contains 4% of w/v formaldehyde. 10% formalin in

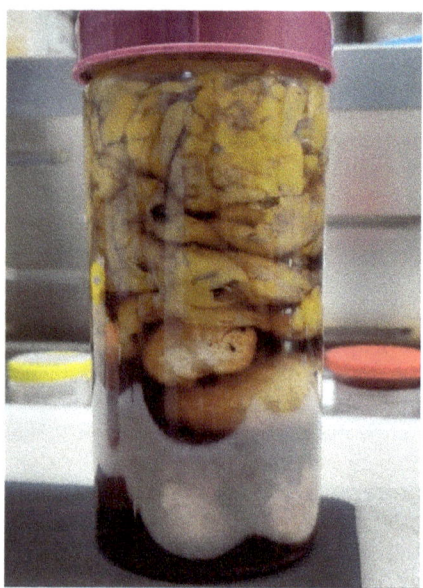

Fig. 6.10: Volume ratio of fixative—Morcellated specimen packed in a bottle. Such specimens should be transferred into wide mouth large container with adequate amount of fixative.

combination with precise concentrations of salts will react well with tissues.

Commercially formalin is available as 37–40% w/v. It is advisable to check concentration of formalin and accordingly dilute formalin to make precise concentration of 10%.

❖ **Osmolality:** Osmolality is salt concentrations in the fixative solution. The osmolality is expressed as Osm. Tonicity refers to the water potential of two solutions separated by a partially permeable membrane. Hypotonic solutions give rise to cell swelling and poor fixation. Hypertonic solution result in cell shrinkage. Slightly hypertonic solution of fixative works best (400–450 mOsm). 0.9% Sodium chloride solution with osmolality 250–300 mOsm is used to maintain the balance in the preparation of 10% formal saline 10% Neutral buffered formalin is highly hypertonic (~18,00 mOsm), most of the tonicity is related to reduced power of formaldehyde molecules due to formation of methylene glycol. Hence buffering with sodium dihydrogen phosphate ($NaH_2PO_4.H_2O$), disodium hydrogen phosphate ($Na_2H_2PO_4$) helps in preserving tissue morphology.

Techniques of Tissue Fixation

- **Fixation by immersion:** Tissue is immersed in a fixative solution in proportion of 20:1.
- **Fixation using perfusion:** This technique is used in research work of animal studies (rat/mice).
- **Fixation by vapor:** Used for demonstration of catecholamines in nervous tissue; tissues are fixed in presence of dry formaldehyde vapor at 60 to 80°C.
- **Coating or spraying fixative:** Used for fixation of cytology smears.

Fixatives as Per their Action on Cells and Tissue

- Microanatomical fixatives preserve the anatomy of tissue; maintain relationship between tissue layers and large aggregates of cells. These fixatives are used in routine histopathology.
- Cytological fixatives are used for preservation of intracellular structures or inclusions that needs to be observed. For details of cytological fixative refer to Cytopathology chapter.

- **Histochemical fixatives:** Freeze drying technique, best example in practice is using cryostat.

Types

- **Physical**
  - *Heat:* Coagulation of proteins and melting of lipids
  - Microwave fixation by stabilizing proteins; speeds fixation
  - *Freeze drying:* This is achieved by immersing tissue in isopentane cooled to its freezing point 170°C using liquid nitrogen.
- **Chemical**
  - *Coagulant fixative:* Fixative that coagulate proteins allows easy sectioning of paraffin embedded tissue but can destroy cytoplasmic organelles as mitochondria, lysozyme, and secretory granules. This group of fixatives act by displacing water from proteinaceous material there by breaking the hydrogen bonds and disturbing tertiary structure to the change known as denaturation. Nucleic acids are not precipitated and remain in the water.

Summary of reagents used as/for fixative		
Coagulant fixative		**Noncoagulant fixative**
Nonadditive	**Additive**	
Alcohols	Mercuric chloride	Formaldehydes
Acetone	Chromic acid	Glutaraldehyde
Acetic acid	Picric acid	Glyoxal
	Cupric salts	Osmium tetroxide
		Potassium dichromate

- *Non-coagulant fixative:* These fixative acts by cross linking the structural macromolecules of the tissue. Cross linking of proteins by converting cytoplasm into gel in which organelles are preserved.

Formaldehyde (CH_2O)

It is a gas which is about 37–40% (by weight) soluble in water. This saturated solution is available commercially as 37–40% (w/v) formaldehyde or formalin. A small amount (10–12%) of methanol is added to supress oxidation and polymerization. 10% formalin is prepared using 1 part of formaldehyde + 9 parts of water and contains 3.7–4.0 % formaldehyde. Formaldehyde is both noncoagulant and an additive fixative. 10% Formalin is commonly used fixative in routine that does not cause excessive tissue shrinkage or distortion of tissue components during fixation.

Mechanism of formalin fixation – Penetration + Crosslinking

Formaldehyde penetrates quickly into the specimen by diffusion to reach innermost layers of the cells. The process involves formation of cross links with proteins groups amines, amides, aromatic amino acid chains sulfhydryl side chains.

Formaldehyde when dissolved in water is hydrated to form methylene glycol because of which tissues when placed in formaldehyde are penetrated rapidly. Methylene glycol hydrate molecules to react with each other combining to form polymers, $H_2C=O + H_2O \rightarrow HOCH_2OH$. At neutral or alkaline pH, it depolymerizes to methylene glycol which dehydrates into carbonyl formaldehyde ($^+CH_2-OH$) which is reactive electrophile form of formaldehyde. This carbonyl formation reacts with various functional groups of macromolecules in a fixation process. The initial crosslinking is completed within 24–48 hours which is reversible. Later due to formation of stable covalent cross linkages after over fixation are not irreversible. The subsequent crosslinking occurs on compound RH+ CH$_2$O → R.CH$_2$(OH) by formation of crosslink of—CH$_2$—a methylene bridge. These methylene bridges can be readily broken by hydrolysis. Only loosely bound formaldehyde can be removed by conventional washing.

The equilibrium between formaldehyde as carbonyl formaldehyde and methylene glycol makes formaldehyde solution penetrate fast and take longer time to fixation of tissue due to effect of polymerization. Hence it is recommended to use freshly prepared solution of formalin which will be of help to keep the concentrations of polymer low.

Mercuric Chloride (HgCl$_2$)

Combines with the acid groups of proteins and the phosphoric groups of nucleoproteins, reacts specifically, with 'SH' group. It is a protein precipitant which rapidly penetrates and hardens. Mercuric chloride containing fixatives are B 5, Zenker's fluid. These were commonly used for fixation of hemopoietic tissues.

Tissues fixed in any mercury containing fixative will require treatment with 0.5% iodine in 70% ethanol for 5–10 minutes to convert it to mercuric iodide and then it is removed by treating with sodium thiosulfate. Due to the inherent toxicity of mercury, these fixatives have been discontinued from most laboratories.

Potassium Dichromate (K$_2$Cr$_2$O$_7$)

It has a binding effect on protein similar to that of formalin. It gives fixation of the cytoplasm without precipitation. The main affinity of chromium ions is for carboxyl and hydroxyl groups of protein and hence it is unsuitable for histochemistry.

Following fixation in potassium dichromate (or chromic acid) tissue must be washed well in running water before dehydration.

Picric Acid ($C_6H_3N_3O_7$)

Picric acid is used as an additive in fixation process. It produces marked cell shrinkages hence not used alone. It precipitates proteins and combines with them to form picrate's. Some of the water-soluble picrate's must be rendered insoluble by treatment with alcohol before the tissue comes in contact with water.

Picric acid has to be stored in a moist, humid place because of its explosive nature.

Ethyl Alcohol

It is mainly used as a fixative for blood films and smears. It penetrates slowly in tissues and hardens the tissue after long exposure. It denatures protein by precipitation and also precipitates glycogen.

It is used in histochemical methods for enzymes since they are left in original state.

It dissolves fats and lipids. Used in Carney's fixative.

Methanol is used for fixation on blood and bone marrow smears.

Glutaraldehyde ($C_5H_8O_2$)

It is principally used in combination with osmium tetroxide for electron microscopy. It reacts chiefly with amino groups. It also reacts with tyrosine, tryptophan, and phenylalanine. It is the most efficient cross-linking agent for collagen. Its cross-linking efficiency gives better preservation of structure and more rapid fixing action than formaldehyde, but poorer penetration.

At pH levels >8.0 it undergoes rapid polymerization.

Osmium Tetra oxide (OsO_4)

It gives excellent preservation of details of minute pieces of tissue or of single cells; hence it is exclusively used in electron microscopy. It demonstrates lipids. It is very expensive and while handling it is necessary to take extra care since its vapors are irritating and may cause conjunctivitis.

Preparation of Fixatives

1. 10% Formalin
   - Formaldehyde (40% w/v)   10 mL
   - Distilled water/RO water   90 mL
2. 10% Buffered formalin
   - Formaldehyde (40% w/v)   100 mL
   - Distilled water/RO water   900 mL
   - Sodium dihydrogen phosphate ($NaH_2PO_4.H_2O$)   4.0 g
   - Disodium hydrogen phosphate ($Na_2H_2PO_4$)   6.5 g

   Note: Buffering capacity means water's ability to keep the pH stable as acid or bases are added to the formaldehyde (40% w/v), a gas available in aqueous solution and unbuffered.
3. 10% Formal saline
   - Formaldehyde (40% w/v)   100 mL
   - Distilled water/RO water   900 mL
   - Sodium chloride   9 g
4. AZF (Acetic zinc formalin)
   - Formaldehyde (40% w/v)   15 mL
   - Zinc chloride   1.25 mL
   - Distilled water   85 mL
   - Glacial acetic acid   0.75 mL

   Ideal for fixation of bone marrow biopsy and lymphoid tissue

5. FAA – Formalin – acetic acid – alcohol

50% (or 70%) Ethanol	90 mL
Glacial acetic acid	0.5 mL
Formaldehyde (40% w/v)	5 mL

Rapid in action; used for fixing MRM specimens; advised to prepare fresh

6. Buffered formal sucrose

Formalin	10 mL
Sucrose	7.5 g
M/15, phosphate buffer (pH 7.4)	100 mL

This is an excellent fixative for the preservation of fine structure, phospholipids, and some enzymes. It is recommended for combined cytochemistry and electron microscopic studies.

It should be used cold (4°C) on fresh tissue.

Mercuric Chloride Containing Fixative

1. Heidenhain Susa

Mercuric chloride	4.5 g
Sodium chloride	0.5 g
Trichloroacetic acid	2.0 g
Acetic acid	4.0 mL
Distilled water	100 mL

Excellent fixative for routine biopsy work. Allows brilliant staining with good cytological detail. Gives rapid and even penetration with minimum shrinkage. Tissues should be treated with iodine to remove mercury pigment.

2. Zenker's fluid

Mercuric chloride	5 g
Potassium dichromate	2.5 g
Sodium sulfate	1.0 g

Distilled water to	100 mL
Just before use add glacial acetic acid	5 mL

Rapid fixation

It is not stable after the addition of acetic acid, hence acetic acid (or formalin) should be added just before use. Washing of tissue in running water is necessary to remove excess dichromate. Mercuric chloride pigment should be removed with iodine.

3. Helly's fluid (Zenker's formal)

Mercuric chloride	5 g
Potassium dichromate	2.5 g
Sodium sulfate	1.0 g
Distilled water to	100 mL
Just before use add formalin	5 mL

An excellent fixative for bone marrow, spleen and blood containing organs.

As with Zenker's fluid it is necessary to remove excess dichromate and mercuric pigment

Picric acid containing fixative –

4. Bouin's fluid

Saturated aqueous picric acid	75 mL
Formalin	25 mL
Glacial acetic acid	5 mL

Rapid fixation, penetrates evenly and causes little shrinkage. Brilliant staining with trichrome stains.

5. Gendre's solution

95% Ethanol saturated with picric acid	800 mL
Formalin	150 mL
Acetic acid	50 mL

Better fixative for glycogen and other carbohydrates. After fixation tissue to be placed in 70% alcohol.

Histochemical Fixatives

The functions of a good histochemical fixative are: (1) preservation of the constituents to be demonstrated (2) preservation of its morphological relationships (3) preservation of the specific tissue constituents and (4) not to affect the reagent to be used in the process of visualization.

For the majority of histochemical methods, *cryostat cut sections* of rapidly frozen tissue or sections of frozen dried tissue are preferred. These sections are used unfixed or fixed by a vapor fixative.

Buffered formalin is the most common fixative used for histochemical purposes. Immersion in *acetone,* 0–4°C is widely used for the fixation of tissues in which it is intended to study enzymes (particularly the phosphatases). The fixation of sections cut from freeze-dried material may be affected by immersion in *absolute alcohol* for 24 hours.

Vapor Fixatives

These are used to fix cryostat cut sections of fresh tissue and sections of blocks of frozen dried tissue. These fixatives are used inside an airtight glass container with controlled heat and humidity to fix *cryostat cut sections* of fresh tissue and sections or blocks of frozen dried tissue.

Following are the various vapor fixatives used in histopathology laboratory.
1. **Formaldehyde:** Paraformaldehyde is heated (50 to 80°C) to obtain vapours. For fixation, blocks of tissue require 3–5 hours and sections require 1/2 to 1 hour at 50–60°C.
2. **Acetaldehyde:** It is used by heating at 80°C for 1–4 hours.

3. **Glutaraldehyde:** A 50% (v/v) aqueous solution of glutaraldehyde can be used at 80°C for 2 minutes to 4 hours or at 60°C for 7 hours.
4. **Acrolein or chromyl chloride:** This reagent is used in liquid form at 37°C for 1–2 hours.

BIBLIOGRAPHY

1. Chemical and physical basics of routine formaldehyde fixation. JOMFP. 2012(Sep-Dec);16(3):400.
2. Formaldehyde Crosslinking: A Tool for the Study of Chromatin Complexes*. JBC. 2015(October 30);290(44):26404-11.
3. Fox CH, Johnson FB, Whiting J, Roller PP. Formaldehyde Fixation. J Histochem Cytochem. 1985; 33:84553.
4. Grizzle WE, Fredenburgh JL, Myers RB. Fixation of tissues. In: Bancroft JD, Gamble M (Eds). Theory and Practice of Histological Techniques. 6th edition. Philadelphia, USA: Elsevier Limited; 2008. p. 5663.
5. https://en.wikipedia.org/wiki/Formaldehyde
6. https://en.wikipedia.org/wiki/Histopathology
7. https://www.cancer.gov/publications/dictionaries/cancer-terms/def

TISSUE PROCESSING AND EMBEDDING

The most common method used for tissue processing is the paraffin wax method. Embedding in paraffin is accomplished most rapidly and gives the best results when thin sections of tissue sections are prepared for viewing under light microscopy. Since paraffin wax was first introduced by Edwin Klebs in 1869 paraffin wax is extensively used as an infiltration and embedding medium.

Since paraffin is not miscible in water tissue processing is designed to remove water and are equilibrated with reagents that are miscible with wax. Specimens adequately fixed and submitted for grossing. Tissue bits are filled in cassettes and submitted for processing.

Tissue sections are also processed using cryostat or freezing microtome for diagnosis purposes.

Tissue processing stages involve

Dehydration—Alcohol

Dehydration is complete removal of water from tissue. This process removes residual fixative and unbound water from the tissue and replace with dehydrating fluid. Alcohol is used with gradual increase in concentration for dehydration. A higher concentration of alcohol in the beginning should be avoided. Rapid removal of water will result in tissue shrinkage.

Incomplete dehydration **(Fig. 6.11)** will not allow infiltration of clearing agent and tissues will remain soft. Excess dehydration will result in hard, shrunken, and brittle tissue.

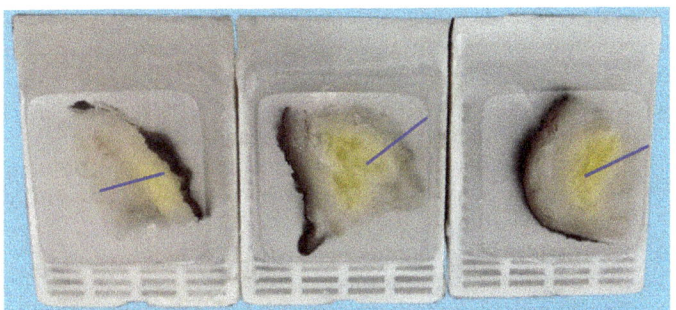

Fig. 6.11: Incomplete fixation and dehydration.

Ethyl alcohol and isopropyl alcohol is of choice for tissue processing. Ethyl alcohol is diluted in sequence with gradual increase for processing starting from 50-60%, 80%, 95% than absolute one. Ethyl alcohol is strictly controlled by the government and available only with license.

Isopropyl alcohol is used directly, without serial dilution for tissue processing. This is an excellent substitute for ethyl alcohol and is easily available for use.

Acetone is used in EM techniques as dehydrating agent. Dioxane and cellosolve are other dehydrating agents.

Note: The reliability of dehydration is checked by using anhydrous copper sulfate (white). The last batch of alcohol is tested with anhydrous copper sulfate. If it turns blue it indicates incomplete dehydration.

Clearing–Xylene

Clearing agent is a fluid that is miscible with both dehydrating and embedding reagent by replacing dehydrating fluid and allowing infiltration by embedding reagent. On completion of the clearing process appearance of tissue is translucent because of refractive index of clearing agents. Excess clearing will result in brittleness to the tissue section.

- Xylene is commonly used as clearing agent.
- Toluene, chloroform, benzene, cedar wood oil can also be used. But Benzene is known carcinogen and cedar wood oil is toxic and more viscous.
- Propylene oxide is clearing agent used in EM.
- Impregnation – **Paraffin wax.**

Paraffin wax is used to support tissue for microtomy. During processing of tissue, the clearing agent xylene is replaced by paraffin wax. During this procedure xylene is eliminated from the tissue by diffusion in the surrounding melted wax (infiltration). The wax afterwards diffuses in the tissue by replacing the xylene (impregnation). The temperature of the paraffin bath should be between 55°C and 60°C. Infiltrated paraffin maintains the intercellular structure during the cutting procedure on microtome.

Paraplast is the mixture of highly purified paraffin wax available in the form of pellets. Different substances can be added to paraffin wax to modify its melting point and consistency which improves its efficiency.

Ceresin, beeswax, microcrystalline wax, bayberry wax were used as additives by increasing hardness of the paraffin wax. With improved consistency of paraffin wax additives are not required in routine however in special techniques and hot weather conditions combination of wax and resin will give best results.

Factors Effecting Tissue Processing
- **Heat:** Increases penetration rate, Care must be taken not to overheat the tissue.
- **Agitation:** Increases flow of reagents around tissue rapid dehydration
- **Vacuum:** Improves impregnation by paraffin wax, by reducing pressure.

Requirements
- Stainless steel or plastic cassettes
- Isopropyl alcohol
- Xylene
- Paraffin wax
- Hot air oven (Temperature 50-60°C)
- Lead pencil and paper
- Cassettes
- Tissue processor

Method

- Tissue blocks are placed in tissue basket after labeling and having entered in gross book.
- The identification number is written with a lead pencil on a piece of paper.
- Tissues are processed as desired.

Before loading tissue processor

- Daily check level of the reagents. Depending upon the utilization of the reagent levelling has to be done.
- Check temperature of paraffin wax bath and to be documented.
- Change of reagent log to be maintained.
- Daily start and finish time of tissue processor to be documented.

For workload of 125 blocks schedule of reagent change -
These are ONLY FOR guidelines FOR DOCUMENTATION

However, schedule can be changed according to the workload and individual laboratory.

1st jar is discarded and added fresh every day	1st jar of isopropyl alcohol is changed alternate day. All jars are taken forward and the last jar of IPA is replaced with fresh.	1st jar of xylene is discarded once a week, the other two jars are taken forward and replaced with fresh xylene in the last jar	Paraffin wax from 1st jar is discarded and 2nd paraffin is kept at 1st position. 2nd Jar is filled with fresh paraffin every 10 to 12 days

Tissue Processing Schedule

Tissues were processed manually till the introduction of automated tissue processor. The technology has evolved gradually.

In the beginning, the tissue processor was designed with the following concepts which availed automatic moment of tissue containing baskets sequentially in the reagent containers overnight processing schedules helped in defining workflow for technical staff.

Open Tissue Processor (Fig. 6.12)

- Perforated baskets and tissue cassettes were designed for processing of tissue samples.
- Number of stations were defined as per manual protocol
- Reagent containers were arranged in circular position
- Action of transfer was designed mechanically for transfer of baskets
- Schedule for processing was defined on the disc connected mechanically to the movement of tissue processor. The processing timing is notched on the disc with timing of 24-hours.
- Immediate/delay start facility
- In case of power failure tissues were able to process manually on the processor using timings of manual processing.

Although these processors helped in processing tissue faster than manual technique without human involvement. These models were further improved with digital facility for defining schedule. However, evaporation of reagents and health hazard with reagent fumes continued as disadvantage.

Technology Further Improved with new Developments

Carousel Type Tissue Processors (Fig. 6.13)

- Rotation, vertical oscillation of the tissue basket
- Vacuum function with fumes control facility controls evaporation of reagents

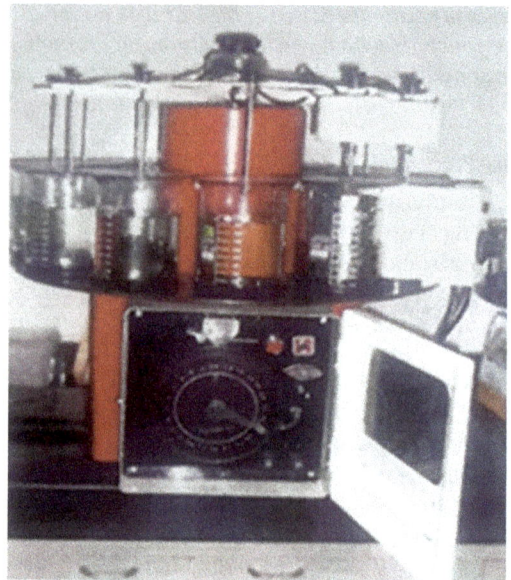

Fig. 6.12: Open tissue processor.

- Programmable spinning speed, if desired spinning can be put off.
- Allowed improvement in dehydration/clearing/impregnation processes by reducing processing timings.
- Reagent carryover reduced due to facility of gentle centrifugal spinning of basket above reagent vessel.
- In case of power failure in built battery backup facility

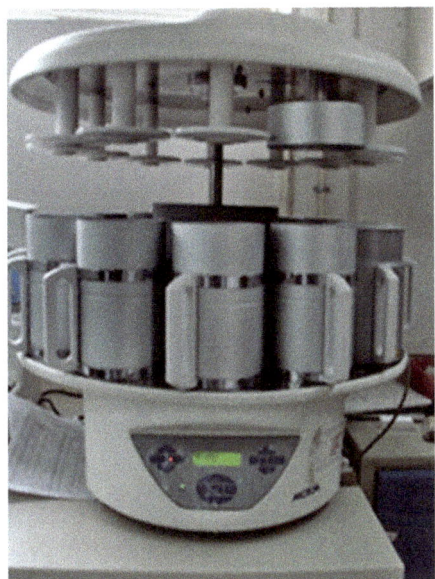

Fig. 6.13: Carousel type processor.

Enclosed Tissue Processors (Fig. 6.14)

Vacuum, heating and bubbling technology are main features.
- In the closed type of systems tissue cassettes remain in the in a closed chamber and reagents are made to flow in and out through their individual pipes.
- Improved quality of tissue processing due to no reagent contamination and less wastage of reagents.

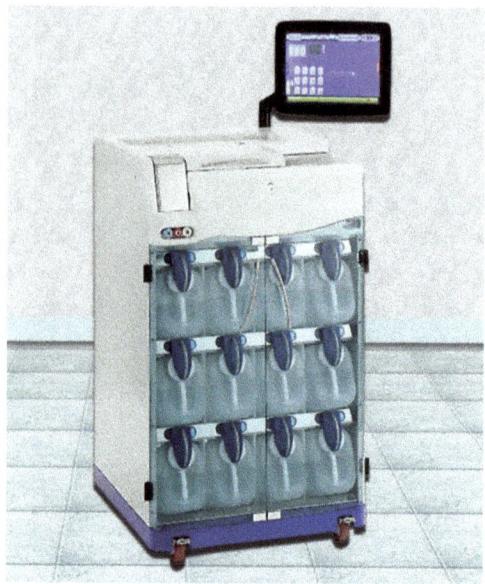

Fig. 6.14: Enclosed tissue processor.

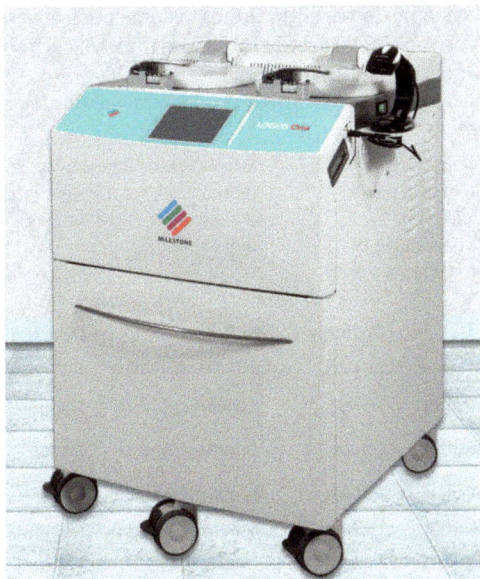

Fig. 6.15: Microwave based rapid tissue processor.

❖ These systems do not allow fumes to come out from equipment. Fumes are being extracted and passed through carbon filter and pure air is circulated in laboratory.

*Processing schedules are defined ONLY as guidelines. Individual laboratory can have their own schedule.

Manual tissue processing method—In case of power failure or equipment breakdown, processing of larger tissue bits is processed manually

Simple tissue processor that functions mechanically for transfer of tissue; tissue processing timing is notched on 24-hour timing disc

Solution	Duration	Solution	Duration
10% Formal saline	2 hours	10% Formal saline	1 hour
Isopropyl alcohol	1 hour	Isopropyl alcohol	1 hour
Isopropyl alcohol	1 hour	Isopropyl alcohol	1 hour
Isopropyl alcohol	2 hours	Isopropyl alcohol	1 hour
Isopropyl alcohol	1½ hour	Isopropyl alcohol	1 hour
Isopropyl alcohol	1½ hour	Isopropyl alcohol	1 hour
Isopropyl alcohol	Overnight	Isopropyl alcohol	1 hour 30 minutes
Xylene I	1 hour	Isopropyl alcohol	1 hour 30 minutes
Xylene II	1 hour	Xylene I	1 hour
Xylene III	1 hour	Xylene II	1 hour
Paraffin wax I	2 hours	Xylene III	1 hour 30 minutes
Paraffin wax II	2 hours	Paraffin wax I	1 hour
		Paraffin wax II	1 hour 30 minutes

A carousel type tissue processor enables rotation/vertical oscillation of the tissue basket. This action helps in improved dehydration/clearing/impregnation processes and reduces processing time. (STP 120, TP 1020, PTO5TS)

Solution	Overnight protocol Duration	Rush biopsy protocol Duration	Oscillation rate
10% Formal saline	1 hour	20 minutes	A1 – 60 rpm
Isopropyl alcohol	1 hour	10 minutes	A1 – 60 rpm
Isopropyl alcohol	1 hour	10 minutes	A1 – 60 rpm
Isopropyl alcohol	1 hour	10 minutes	A1 – 60 rpm
Absolute isopropyl alcohol I	1 hour	15 minutes	A1 – 60 rpm
Absolute isopropyl alcohol II	1 hour	10 minutes	A1 – 60 rpm
Absolute isopropyl alcohol III	1 hour	15 minutes	A1 – 60 rpm
Xylene I	1 hour	10 minutes	A1 – 60 rpm
Xylene II	1 hour	15 minutes	A1 – 60 rpm
Xylene III	1 hour	15 minutes	A1 – 60 rpm
Paraffin wax I	1 hour 30 minutes	30 minutes	A2 – 70 rpm
Paraffin wax II	1 hour 30 minutes	30 minutes	A2 – 70 rpm

The enclosed tissue processor has facility of vacuum, heating and bubbling technology. All these 3 technologies help in superior impregnation of reagent in tissues compared to carousel open tissue processor. (EFTP, Leica Histo core Pearl)

Solution	Overnight protocol Time in minutes	Rush biopsy protocol Time in minutes	Temp °C	PV	MX
10% NBF	60	0	Ambient	NO P/V	2
70% Isopropyl alcohol	60	20	Ambient	V	2
80% Isopropyl alcohol	60	20	Ambient	V	2
90% Isopropyl alcohol	60	20	Ambient	V	2
90% Isopropyl alcohol	60	20	Ambient	V	2
Absolute isopropyl alcohol I	60	20	Ambient	V	2
Absolute isopropyl alcohol II	60	20	Ambient	V	2
Absolute isopropyl alcohol III	60	20	Ambient	V	2
Xylene I	60	20	30	V	2
Xylene II	60	20	30	V	2
Xylene III	60	20	30	V	2
Paraffin wax I	60	20	60	NO P/V	2
Paraffin wax II	60	20	60	V	2

Xylene being hazardous reagent however most popular clearing agent used in techniques of histopathology.

Need of hour—Xylene free protocol

Study was conducted at Bronson Methodist Hospital using Leica PELORIS tissue processor. Reagents used were ethanol and isopropyl alcohol. Leica has introduced Paralast as xylene substitute for processing. This protocol is applicable on enclosed tissue processor only. Miniscule amount of xylene is only used for cleaning and maintenance of equipment.

Xylene free protocol					
	1.11-hour Protocol		12.1-hour Protocol		PV
Solution	Temp °C	Time in minutes	Temp °C	Time in minutes	
10% NBF	37	15	37	60	-
Processing water (D/W)	-	02	-	02	-
Isopropyl alcohol I	45	05	45	60	-
Isopropyl alcohol II	45	05	45	60	-
Isopropyl alcohol III	50	05	50	60	-
Isopropyl alcohol IV	50	05	50	60	-
Isopropyl alcohol V	50	05	50	60	-
Isopropyl alcohol VI	50	10	50	60	-
Paralast	60	04	60	04	-
Paraffin wax I	65	05	65	90	V
Paraffin wax II	65	05	65	90	V
Paraffin wax III	65	05	65	120	V

Microwave based tissue processor **(Fig. 6.15)**– *Logos introduced by milestone.*

Ultra-rapid dehydration/clearing steps are carried out by microwave heating technology allows faster turnaround time. Xylene

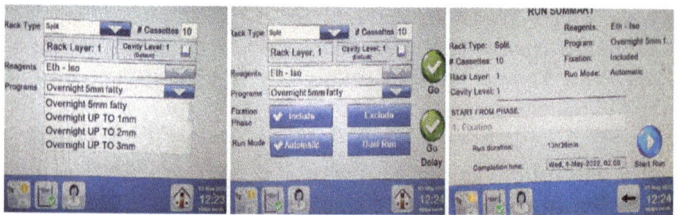

Fig. 6.16: In built tissue processing schedule.

free protocol uses combination of alcohol and isopropyl alcohol for processing. This equipment has inbuilt programs defined as per specimen thickness **(Fig. 6.16)**.

Equipment has facility to run multiple batches for processing during the day.

Specimen thickness	Rapid protocol
<1 mm; Transplant biopsy	Full batch* processed in 34 minutes (including fixation)
1 mm (GI/endoscopic biopsies)	Full batch processed in 1 h 40 minutes (including fixation)—210 cassettes
1 mm (GI/endoscopic biopsies)	Full batch processed in 1 h 40 minutes (including fixation)—140 cassettes
3 mm	Full batch** processed in 3 h 5 minutes (including fixation)
5 mm	Full batch** processed in 5 h 56 minutes (including fixation)

*Up to 70 cassettes **Up to 140 cassettes with 1-gallon containers and up to 210 cassettes with 5 liter reagent jars

Re-Processing of Tissues

In case of bad fixation, bad processing, equipment failure tissues can be reprocessed back.

Method

1. Tissue is removed off paraffin block by placing in the oven at 60°C.
2. Tissue bits are transferred in a cassette and submitted for reprocessing.
3. Transfer cassettes in:
   - Two changes of xylene for 1 hour each. Check for tissue appearance.
   - Two changes of isopropyl alcohol for 1 hour each.
   - Wash under running tap water
   - Submit back in routine processing schedule
4. Incomplete decalcification tissues can be processed again—
   - Bring tissue back to running tap water.
   - Place tissue in decalcifying solution (10% nitric acid)
   - On completion of decalcification wash tissue in water for 4–6 hours
   - Submit back in routine processing schedule

Document reprocessing data with corrective and preventive action.

Tissue Embedding

Embedding enables the tissue to be cut on a microtome.

After infiltration by warm liquid paraffin wax specimens are unloaded for tissue processor for embedding. Embedding is defined as blocking or casting of tissue in warm liquid paraffin which forms firm block after cooling. Embedding is done by filling a metal base mold of suitable size with molten paraffin. Tissues are oriented in the base mold ensuring that its being cut in the right plane. A plastic holder is put over the mold and it is allowed to solidify. Cut surface of tissue rests flat on the base of mold. After cooling metal mold is peeled away and plastic holder remains attached to paraffin block. The paraffin block with holder can be directly clamped on to the microtome.

In earlier days wooden blocks or metal holders were attached to paraffin blocks and then were used to clamped on to microtome for cutting. Now plastic embedding rings and embedding cassettes are used as holder.

Embedding Molds

For embedding process techniques have evolved from manual to tissue embedding systems.

For block making—paper boats, ice trays, Leukhartz 'L' brass molds **(Fig. 6.17)**, Tissue Tek base **(Fig. 6.18)** molds.

Holders for microtome attachment **(Fig. 6.19)**-Wooden block metal holders and plastic holders by Tissue Tek.

Base molds

Leukhartz mold, 'L' shaped embedding mold is made up of two 'L' shaped pieces of heavy metallic brass.

Tissue Tek molds are used as base molds. They are made up of stainless steel and are available in different sizes, 7 × 7 mm, 15 × 15 mm, 24 × 24 mm, 37 × 24 mm

Paraffin block holder

Wooden block, metal holders, plastic rings, tissue tek holder (embedding cassettes)

Fig. 6.17: For block making—paper boats, ice trays, Leukhartz 'L' brass molds.

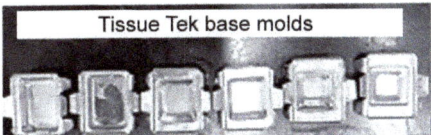

Fig. 6.18: Tissue Tek base molds.

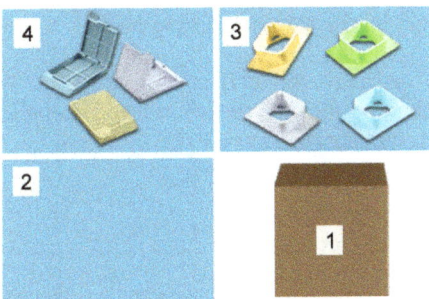

Fig. 6.19: Holders for microtome attachment: (1) Wooden block; (2) Metal holder; (3) Plastic ring; (4) Tissue Tek holder.

Tissue embedding system (Fig. 6.20) is combination of the following:
- wax dispenser
- Wax reservoir, 3–5 liter capacity
- Cold plate (−5 to +5°C) temperature, 50 to 60°C

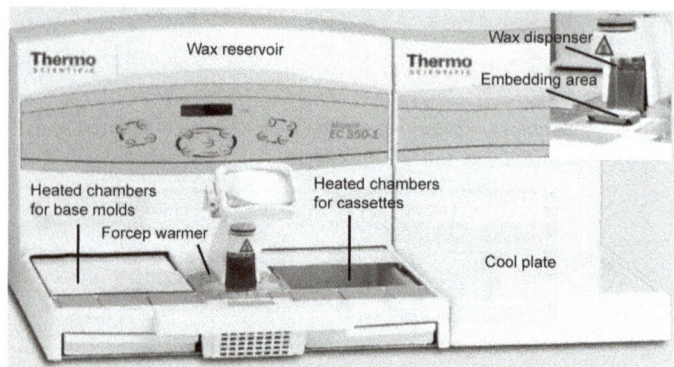

Fig. 6.20: Embedding station.

- 60 blocks can be placed on it for cooling
- Heated chambers for storage of moulds, forceps. Cassettes
- Cold plate adjusted to −5 to + 5°C
- Drain tray for excess wax

Advantages of the systems are
- Easy to operate, reduces labor
- Improves speed for embedding
- Facility for orientation of tissue—lens view for biopsies, cool and warm plate in embedding area

Method

Prerequisite for manual embedding
- Forceps
- Paraffin wax
- Container for warming wax
- Small jug for pouring wax

- Spirit lamp
- Gauze piece

Note: Fill the container with paraffin wax allow it to melt in hot air oven

- **Embedding using "L" molds:** *Traditional embedding method* "L" molds are placed on glass plate. The two "L" pieces are joined to form a side of the rectangular box that acts as a cast to make the mould. Glycerin may be applied to the glass and "L" pieces. Molten paraffin wax is poured in the mould. Tissue is oriented in the mold using warm forcep; label is placed on it; this is allowed to cool. On cooling molds are separated. Wax is cut into different blocks to separate tissues. Wooden blocks or metal holder is attached to the block. Now paraffin block is ready for microtomy. In case of large workload multiple "L" molds are placed on the glass plate and blocking is done.
- Plastic embedding rings were in practice along with introduction of stainless-steel base mold. The tissue is placed in the base of mold plastic ring is placed on it. Wax is poured in the ring and cooled. Plastic acts as a block holder.
- **Embedding cassette as holder:** This is modification of plastic embedding ring. These cassettes are used for processing of tissue. Hence labeling is done at the time of processing. The base of the cassette has one end with slope on which identification number is written. This helps to overcome the labeling errors.

For embedding cassette is opened and base of the cassette is used as holder during embedding.

Tissue Embedding Process

- Remove tissue cassettes from tissue processor and place on the hot plate.
- Open one cassette at a time; open the lid. Discard lid aside.

- Select base mold of appropriate size for tissue to be placed in comfortably.
- Dispense small amount of melted paraffin in the mould. Using clean and slightly warm forceps to pick up the tissue and place it into the wax in the mold. Place the plane to be cut facing downward. Gently press the tissue down with forceps.
  Care must be taken to prevent contamination of samples in embedding step.
- Place the cassette base on top of the mold, add paraffin wax to fill the mold make sure that no bubbles are formed.
- Move the mold to the tray for cooling.
- Once the blocks have cooled, pop them out of the molds with a knife and scrape if any residual paraffin from the sides before proceeding to cutting.

Guidelines for Orientation of Tissue (Figs. 6.21A to D)

- Use appropriate size of base mold for embedding.
- Embed tissue in the center of mold; leave at least 1mm of paraffin wax on the sides which will allow paraffin wax to support for the tissue while sectioning.

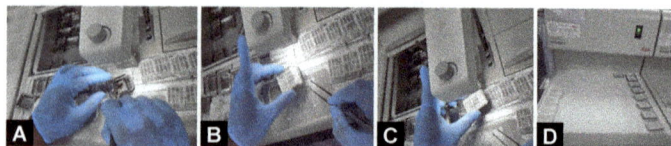

Figs. 6.21A to D: Steps of orientation of tissue: (A) Mold is kept on small cool area. Tissue is oriented immediately in the mold when wax at base is semi solid; (B) Plastic ring is placed over the mold with label added on it; (C) Plastic ring is filled with wax; (D) Plastic is allowed to cool on cooling plate.

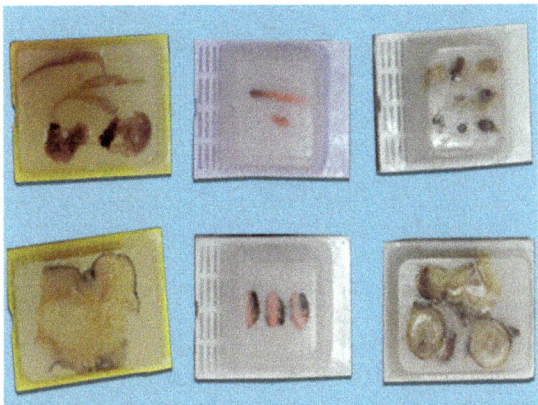

Fig. 6.22: Embedding images: Membrane, bone marrow multiple bits. Skin, inked tissue, tubular structure.

- Place multiple tissue fragments **(Fig. 6.22)** uniformly and quickly before paraffin wax is solidified.
- Bone marrow, Tru-cut needle biopsies must be placed horizontally.
- Muscle tissue to be embedded in both planes, transverse and longitudinal.
- Any tubular structure such as fallopian tubes, appendix to be embedded transversely **(Fig. 6.23)**
- Skin biopsies, cyst walls, ovarian cyst is to be tissue oriented in vertical upright position.
- Inked tissue or margins are embedded oriented by placing inked surface downwards.
- Endoscopic biopsy is placed in a way that all mucosal layers can be viewed.

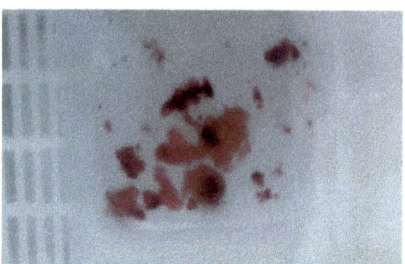

Fig. 6.23: Multiple bits unevenly spread.

Precautions to avoid errors during embedding—
- Paraffin wax should be clean and dust free.
- Temperature of paraffin wax to be monitored strictly and document in the log.
- Open one cassette at a time to avoid mix-up.
- To avoid floaters in tissue sections, clean the forceps in between two blocks.
- At the end of embedding check for the blocks made with actual number of cassettes from tissue loading register, in case of any discrepancy check with concerned staff and document in the error log.

Quality Check:
- Evaluate quality of embedding during sectioning of paraffin block.
- Tissue pieces should be embedded on the same plane.
- There should be no bubbles in the block.
- Specimens must be oriented properly.

If there are issues with embedding, the block should be melted by warming it in a mold and then re-embedded and to be documented in the log.

Problems in Tissue Processing

- ❖ **Electric failure:** Machine will get stuck
  - UPS back up is necessary for the tissue processor
- ❖ **Equipment failure**
  - *Machine skips station*—mechanical problem
    - Inform service engineer
    - *Machine gets stuck up*—restart machine
    - *In formalin jar*—restart machine
    - *In alcohol*—check for completion of dehydration and proceed for clearing
    - *In xylene*—check for completion of clearing and transfer in paraffin
  - *Temperature of paraffin wax bath*
    - Paraffin wax bath have thermostat control in case of failure wax will solidify
    - Wax bath need to be sent for repair
    - It is ideal to have spare wax bath as back up
- ❖ Floaters are small bits of tissue seen on the slide which belongs to other tissue.
  - Floaters arise from messy procedures on the gross table, gloves, gross equipment
    - It is essential to gross one specimen at a time, clean thoroughly before opening another specimen.
  - Tissues also can be transferred as floaters from reusable cassettes if they are not cleaned properly. During embedding the forceps can be cause for floaters.
- ❖ Labeling errors can arise due to mistakes in specimen identification
  - Specimen labels can fall off during processing
  - Mislabelling of the specimen—avoid accessioning identical specimen in a series

- Due to mechanical failure tissue basket is hung for long time outside the solution.

❖ Due to mechanical failure if tissue basket is hung for long time outside the solution—during all cassettes are not dipped remain uncovered. Tissues are dried up. These tissues can be restored to a certain extent by rehydration method. Tissues are placed in solution for 18 to 24 hours after which tissues are processed from dehydration stage.

70% Ethanol	70 mL
Glycerol	30 mL
Dithionite	1 g

Use pre coated slides for preparation of tissue sections.

In case of equipment failure document errors with corrective/preventive action (CAPA).

Section Cutting—Microtomy

Introduction

Microtomy is mechanical science by means of which tissue is cut into thin sections, these are stained and observed under microscope. Most of the microtomy is performed on paraffin wax embedded tissue.

The first instrument used for microtomy is known as microtome. The word microtome by Greek definition is *"mikros" meaning small, temnein meaning "to cut"*

First microtome by Cummings (1770) used a wooden device with a slot allotted to accommodate specimen and the razor blade were used for cutting. Charles Chevalier named the cutting device as "Microtome" (1825). A microtome is a mechanical instrument designed for cutting of tissue. The first microtomes suitable for sectioning animal tissues was constructed in 1848, with the popular Cambridge Rocker (1885), Minot (1886), and

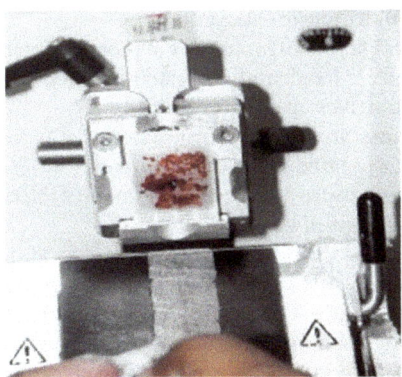

Fig. 6.24: Microtome.

sledge microtomes (1910) manufactured later. Thought process of Rudolf Thoma Heidelberg pathologist and Rudolf Jung precision engineer pioneered journey of series of modern microtomes. It made possible to cut thin uniform sections for microscopic study.

The basic instrument used in microtomy is known as microtome **(Fig. 6.24)**.

The cutting tool is clamped within the instrument. These machines have the facility that will advance an object for a predetermined distance then slide the object to the cutting tool usually knife or blade and force the object through the knife or blade thus producing section. Blocks are chilled prior to cutting. Sections are cut at 3–5 µm with the use of an automatic or manual microtome and mounted onto a pre cleaned glass slide.

Embedded tissues are cut by either a *rotary microtome, rocking microtome* or by a *sliding microtome*. For rotary and rocking microtome, paraffin embedding is required while celloidin-embedded sections are cut by a sliding microtome.

- **Rocking microtome:** Oldest design
  - Cambridge rocking microtome most popular microtome
  - The knife is fixed, and the specimen block moves through arc and strikes against the knife
  - Thickness at which section has to cut is adjusted using ratchet operated micrometer thread
  - Steady backward and forward moment of the handle enables good ribbons of the section.

  Heiffor knife is used. The mechanism is simple and easy to maintain. Knife clamp, block holder, operating handle, micrometer adjustments are unique features of rocking microtome. The term 'rocking' arrives from rocking movement of cross arm. In emergency using ethyl chloride spray can be adapted to use for frozen sections too.

- **Rotary rocking microtome:** Named after its inventor professor Minot as Minot microtome; used for sectioning paraffin blocks; more commonly used in cryostats. While sectioning specimen block moves up and down in vertical plane facing knife with the help of 360-degree rotary movement of the hand wheel.

- **Sliding microtome:** The knife moves horizontally on fixed specimen block. This microtome was developed to use for celloidin embedded tissue blocks.

- **Freezing microtome:** This microtome is clamped to the bench top and is connected to liquid CO_2 cylinder for freezing tissue sample. Updated version of freezing microtome is called cryostat.

- **Base sledge microtome:** Designed for cutting sections of very large blocks. Heavy, stable microtome. The knife or blade is fixed and the specimen block slides under it during sectioning.

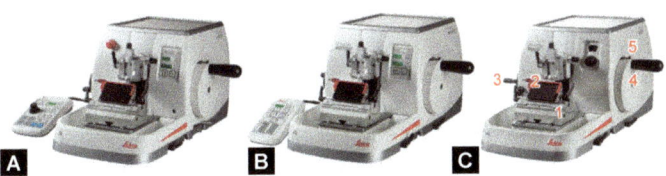

Figs. 6.25A to C: (A) Fully automated; (B) Semi–automated; (C) Manual.

- **Ultra-microtome:** Used for sectioning in electron microscopy.
- **Rotary microtome:** Most commonly used in routine for cutting paraffin wax sections in histopathology laboratory.
- This group of microtomes are available in three types:
    1. *Manual rotary microtome (Fig. 6.25A):* Completely operated by user.
    2. *Semi-automated rotary microtome (Fig. 6.25B):* Automation is introduced for moving of coarse hand wheel
    3. *Fully automated rotary microtome (Fig. 6.25C):* Automation enables both fine and coarse hand wheel; motorized push button sectioning.

Important parts of microtome:
1. Knife holder base
2. Knife holder, 2 in 1 blade holder
3. Coarse hand wheel
4. Advancement of hand wheel
5. Safety Lock

Important features of microtome
- The basic instrument is designed to cut 1 to 60 μ thin sections.
- This instrument possesses cutting tool mechanism for advancement of an object with predetermined distance

and sliding object against knife/blade resulting in thin sections.
- **Specimen retraction facility:** Specimen retraction is to prevent the knife or blade from touching the overlapped specimen while returning to the upper end position, the specimen is retracted 40 μm when retraction is activated. This facility is very important to avoid accidents while sectioning.
- **The block holder:** This holds specimen block in position.
- **Knife holder base:** This is attached on the microtome stage. This can be moved towards or away from paraffin block attached but must be stationary when sectioning is ON.
- **Knife holder:** This is comprised of blade clamp that holds blade, the knife tilt to adjust cutting angle, face plate on which ribbons are passed towards operator.
- **Coarse hand wheel:** Moves forward and backward; used for rough cutting/trimming of sample.
- **Advancement hand wheel:** Turns in one direction at specified/defined microns.
- **Safety lock:** Handwheel locking facility; This prevents moving of wheel when microtome is not in use. Ensure to lock microtome while inserting block/changing blade/cleaning of microtome.

Microtome Knives

Microtome knives are used to cut uniform thin serial tissue sections. Knives can be made of,
- **Metal:** Standard steel, razor blade
- **Non-metal:** Glass, diamond

Classification of based on edge of knife

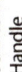
Planoconcave (a, b)

- One side is flat the other concave with different degrees.
- The Plane's surface is close to tissue block.
- Sledge type and certain rotary type of microtome.
- Used for celloidin work

Biconcave

- Concavity on both sides and is designed for cutting paraffin sections on rocking and sledge-type microtome
- Length 10–25 cm

Plane Wedge

- Standard profile
- Types of knives are used for cutting Frozen sections and ordinary paraffin sections.
- Length 10–35 cm
- Wedge knife with deep cutting edge
- Stouter to give rigidity for cutting hard objects
- Available with varying length–freezing microtome 8 cm, base sledge microtome 24 cm

The Heiffor knife—It is used on rocking microtome with a fixed handle

Parts of microtome knife:
- Heel
- Toe—Angle formed by cutting edge
- Honing guide—Also referred as knife back. Each knife has its own back. Back cannot be interchanged
- Handle

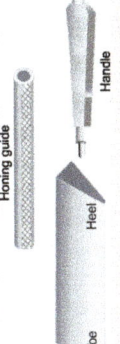

Diamond knife:
- Used for cutting epoxy resin sections electron microscopy
- Cutting edge is of 3 mm
- Very expensive

Knife Sharpening

In the early days the sharpening of knife used to be a manually. Automatic knife sharpeners are now available for sharpening.

Manual sharpening involves two steps—honing and stropping
1. **Honing is process for removing nicks:** Naturally available slabs of stone which had abrasive properties are used for honing.

    Oil is smeared on the surface of stone. Hold knife between thumb and fingers. The knife is diagonally moved forward and backward on stone heel to toe. The cutting edge of the knife must be away from hand facing outward. The movement is continued till nicks are removed. There is no hard and fast rule for time required for honing.

    Common oil used for honing mineral oil, clove oil, xylene, liquid paraffin, soapy water.
2. **Stropping is polishing of knife:** Leather strips are used for stropping. Best strops are made from the rump of horse. The back of the belt is made of canvas. 15–20 stokes are adequate for stropping. Excess strokes can spoil the knife edge. The knife is held with forefinger and thumb, with cutting edge facing inward. It is moved diagonally backward and forward.

Automatic Knife Sharpener (Figs. 6.26A and B)

This is an automatic machine used for knife sharpening. Different models are available—semi-automatic and automatic.

Advantages
1. Sharpens fast
2. Safe operation

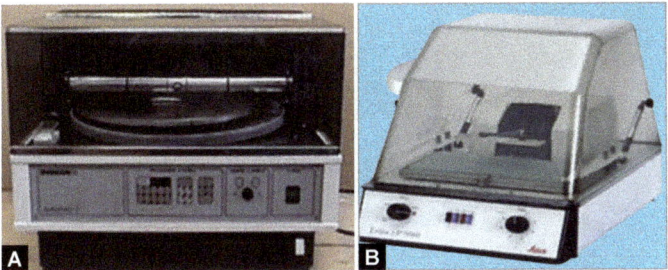

Figs. 6.26A and B: Automatic knife sharpener: (A) Shandon; (B) Leica.

Two types of abrasives were used for sharpening—Coarse and Fine.

Coarse lapping compound consisting of alumina suspension fluid and water is used first followed by compound containing a finer grade of alumina. Lastly, the suspension fluid is used alone to polish the edge.

Maintenance of Microtome Knife

- ❖ The knife must be cleaned with xylene after and before use.
- ❖ When not in use it must be kept in the knife box.
- ❖ Separate knife must be used for bony specimens.
- ❖ Knife must be greased with oil if not being used for long time.

Disposable Knives

Introduction of disposable blades has enabled thin uniform good quality sections and eased the process of sectioning of paraffin block for technical staff. These disposable blades allow flaw less 2–4 µm sections and are used in routine microtomy and in cryostat also. The blades are coated with PTFE (poly tetrafluoroethylene).

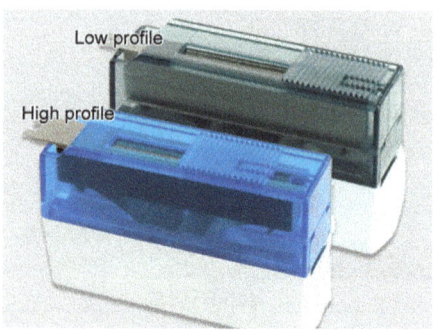

Fig. 6.27: Disposable blades.

These blades are available as low profile and high profile (**Fig. 6.27**) are consistently adaptable for paraffin sections. Separate adapter is required in the microtome for attachment of blades.

Advantages

More convenient to use
- Sharpening is not needed
- Rust free and corrosion resistant edge.

Knife Angle for Microtomy (Fig. 6.28)

The knife plays most important role in producing good sections. Hence the knife should be sharp and well adjusted. Knife angle is also important for thin uniform sections. Correct angle reduces friction preventing compression of the section. Angle of clearance is angle formed between knife edge and paraffin block. It is around 2 to 5° for paraffin sections and 5 to 7° for frozen sections. This will help to avoid friction between knife and block. Clearance angle is angle formed by a line drawn along the block surface and the lower bevel of the knife.

Chapter 6: Histopathology (Prelude to Immunohistochemistry)

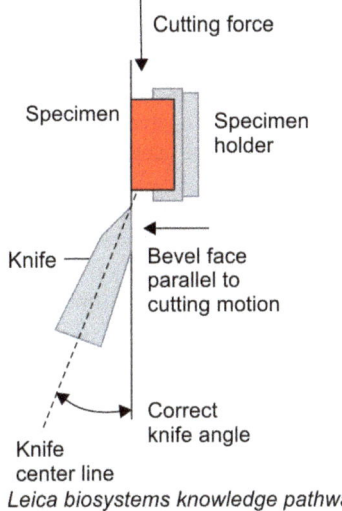

Fig. 6.28: Knife angle for microtomy.

Bevel angle forms by convergence of two planes. It varies from 18°–35°. Angle between the two facets that from the cutting edge. The width of the two facets which makes the cutting edge of knife has recommended from 0.1 to about 0.6 mm.

Slide Adhesives

Paraffin sections are attached to slides in several ways. Sections are dried in oven for attachment and deparaffinization. On few occasions such as staining with strong alkali solutions, tissue containing lots of hemorrhages, cryostat sections used for ancillary stains such as, immunohistochemistry.

Immunofluorescence sections are to be collected on coated slides.

Protein adhesives such as egg albumin and gelatin can be used as adhesive. They are preserved by adding thymol crystals which prevent bacterial overgrowth. However, it needs to be monitored. Adhesives other than protein are used routinely.

- Mayer's egg albumin
    - Equal amount of fresh egg white and glycerol
    - Mix thoroughly. Add thymol crystals as a preservative. Store the stock in refrigerator.
    - A small drop of egg albumin is smeared on the side prior to use.
- Chrome alum—gelatin
    - Gelatin   1.5 g
    - Chromium Potassium sulfate   0.5 g
    - Distilled water   100 mL
    - Gelatin is dissolved in distilled water heated at 60°C. Mix using stirrer until completely dissolved. Mix chromium potassium sulfate into the solution. Add thymol crystals as fixative.
- Poly-L-lysine – Used as 0.1% solution.
- APES, 3-aminopropyltriethoxysilane—2% solution in acetone. Charged slides or plus slides, slides are coated with basic polymer are attached with silicon atoms of the glass.

Note: Slides are cleaned thoroughly with weak acid solutions then rinsed in distilled water at least with two to three changes. Thereafter are dipped in adhesive solution and allowed to dry. These slides are stored in a covered box.

Requirements

- Disposable blades
- **Tissue floatation bath (Fig. 6.29):** A thermostatically controlled water bath is used for floating tissue ribbons after sectioning.

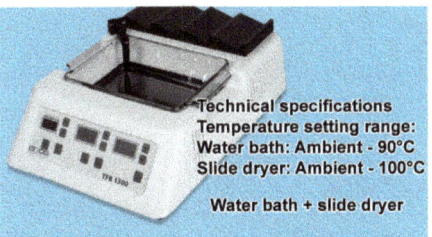

Fig. 6.29: Tissue floatation bath.

The temperature of the water in the bath should be 10°C below the melting point of the paraffin to be sectioned. Care should be taken to prevent water bubbles from being trapped under the section. This can be accomplished by using distilled water in the bath. Alcohol or a small drop of detergent may be added to the water to reduce the surface tension, allowing the section to flatten out with greater ease.

- **Hot air oven or hot plate:** User for drying slides prior to staining for section adhesions. The temperature setting should be approximately that of the melting point of the paraffin. Drying times vary depending on the type of tissue, the number of slides to be dried and size of the drying device. Many automated stainers have drying ovens as part of the instrument, so the time and temperature is easily regulated.

  If the oven is too hot there may be distortion to the cells, causing dark pyknotic nuclei or nuclear bubbling; cells that are completely devoid of nuclear detail.

- Forceps, Brushes, Teasing needles are helpful in the removal of folds, creases and bubbles that may for during floating sections in the floatation bath. Also are useful in picking sections across the knife edge.

- Scalpel
- Slide rack
- Blotting paper
- Ice tray
- Slides
- Slide adhesives
- Lead pencil/diamond pencil

Method

- Fill the water bath with water and turn on water bath to reach desired temperature. (Range of 50 to 55°C).
- Scrape excess paraffin from the cassettes.
- Cool paraffin blocks before cutting.
- Check microtome setting. The blade holder should be adjusted to optimize the clearance angle, the distance between the lower facet angle and the surface of paraffin block. Clamps and screws can be firmly tightened. Place disposable (Low profile) blade in the holder. Care must be taken while placing the blade in the holder, if over tightened can result in uneven tissue sections.
- Sectioning **(Fig. 6.30)**:
    - *Trimming:* Rough cut the PARAFFIN BLOCK by manually advancing using coarse feed mechanism OR by setting microtome at 15–20 μm until entire surface of tissue is exposed.
    - Place the paraffin blocks to be sectioned on cold plate or ice tray in order
    - Ribbons of tissue are produced by making complete revolutions of the cutting wheel.
    - Revolutions should be made at a slow and even speed. This can be controlled by using the keypads on the left side of

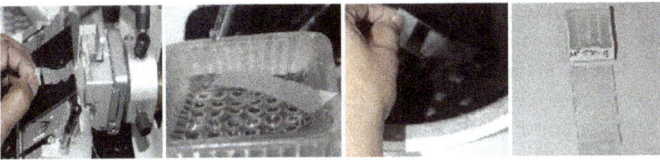

Fig. 6.30: Section is cut; spread well using forceps floated on water bath; picked up on slide; blotted to remove excess water.

the microtome. Wipe away any excess paraffin between taking sections.
- Place the ribbon onto the water bath.
- Using a lead pencil, mark the glass slide with the sample identification number.
- Now select and remove a section from the ribbon. Place the section onto the slide. Remove any bubbles or wrinkles with a camel hairbrush or teasing needle.
- A good section is free of wrinkles, folds, or bubbles.
- Drain excess water by tilting slide onto blotting paper.
- Slides are placed on hot plate (at 60°C) for 2–3 minutes and heated in hot air oven for 10 minutes.
- Slides are now ready to stain.

Once sectioning of all blocks is complete, carefully remove blade from holder and discard into sharps container or into the used blade slot in the blade dispenser. Wipe excess paraffin from microtome and work area. Perform microtome maintenance when required, according to manufacturer's recommendations.

Care and Maintenance of Microtome

Once sectioning of all blocks is complete, carefully remove blade from holder and discard into sharps container or into the used blade slot in the blade dispenser. Wipe excess paraffin from microtome and work area.

Keep the moving parts of the microtome lubricated and clean. The surface should be cleaned frequently.

After cutting sections, accumulated paraffin and tissue should be removed by using a soft brush.

Clean the metal parts carefully with xylene.

Guidelines for Preparing Number of Slides While Sectioning

- All paraffin blocks are routinely cut at 3–4 µm; lymph node, bone marrow biopsy, renal biopsy are cut at 2–3 µm; special stains such as for amyloid or histochemical stains for nerves are to be cut at 6–10 µm.
- Routinely one slide is made from each paraffin block for H&E staining. For anticipated special stains, if noted on worksheet extra slide has to be made for each stain. For example, bone marrow biopsy, renal biopsy, liver biopsy.
- Any additional special stains besides this routine or any deeper sections is to be cut on the next working day.
- Use positively charged slides for Immunohistochemistry work up.

Guidelines for Corrective Action for Problems During Section Cutting

- Tissue sections when floated in warm water sections get disseminated in the water to the extent of No use.
    - *Incomplete impregnation process:* Reprocess tissue.
    - *Water bath temperature is too high:* Monitor temperature of water bath.
- **Thick and thin (uneven) sections:** Paraffin falls on stage while sectioning can lead to instances of grazing the stage.
    - Clean stage in between cutting.

- **Incorrect knife angle:** Adjust knife angle.
- Compressed sections, chatters in section, curling of sections.
- **Blunt knife/blade:** Replace with new blade.
- Chatters in the sections can be reduced by precooling paraffin block, slowing rotation of microtome handle speed.

Section cutting skills can be developed with adequate training and experience. Knowledge of equipment is mandatory. Refer to instructions provided in the technical manual supplied with instrument.

Frozen Section

The concept evolved by Dr Louis B Wilson in 1905. He used Spencer automatic microtome with CO_2 attachment for freezing tissue section. He used dye methylene blue for the staining purpose. He provided the diagnosis to the surgeon within 5 minutes. He experimented and standardized technique of freezing, cutting and staining procedures. Introduction of fluorescent antibody technique in 1941 by Coons et. al., necessitated need of 3-5 μm thin fresh frozen sections. This was permitted by introduction Cryostat in 1954. Preparation of frozen section became easy with the introduction of cryostat with the cabinet cooled to –20 to –30°C and enclosing microtome within.

Frozen section technique is widely used in routine for rapid diagnosis during operation. When tissue is frozen the water contents of tissue section turn to ice and in this state, tissue is firm. Ice acts as an embedding medium.

Applications of Frozen Section

Intraoperative diagnosis for surgical specimens involve:
- Tumor identification
- Resection margin clearance

- Identify metastasis
- Sentinel Lymph node

Other than rapid diagnosis use of frozen sections is used for following:
- Immunofluorescent techniques for kidney, skin biopsies
- Enzyme histochemistry—enzyme activity cannot with stand routine tissue processing
- Demonstration of fat

Specimen

Fresh tissue is received for frozen section. Specimens are received from operation theatre, OPD, radiology department.

Tissue must not be transferred on the gauze piece as water content will be absorbed in the gauze. Specimen must reach the laboratory as soon as possible to avoid drying artifacts.

In institutions cryostat is usually placed in the operation theatre premises.

All specimens received for frozen sections are to be considered as potentially *Dangerous*. Use of PPE apron, gloves, masks are mandatory while handling specimens for frozen.

Grossing of Specimen

As soon as specimen is accessioned and received to be sent for grossing.

Specimen embedding—Select appropriate size of chuck (**Fig. 6.31**). Add cryo compound/water on the chuck.

Place tissue on it. Water content within tissue in addition also helps in hardening tissue. Cryo compound or water act as embedding medium.

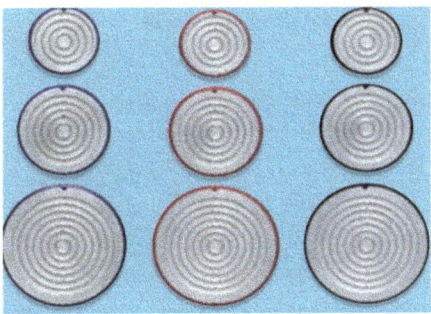

Fig. 6.31: Chucks–metal disc with gripping grid pattern allowing space for tissue and cryomedium to embed firmly.

Cryostat temperature
- Electronic temperature controls up to –35°C
- Cryostat chamber temperature –20° to –25°C

Specimen temperature
Depending on the nature of the tissue the temperature is decided for freezing
- Lymph node, liver, kidney, spleen, thyroid –12° to –16°C
- Breast, skin, muscle –20° to –30°C

Cryostat (**Fig. 6.32**) is a freezer containing microtome. The type of microtome used is rotary type. It serves the purpose of quick freezing and subsequent sectioning of the tissue.

Cryostat Disinfection

All specimens received for frozen section are considered as potentially dangerous hence maintaining good hygiene of cryostat

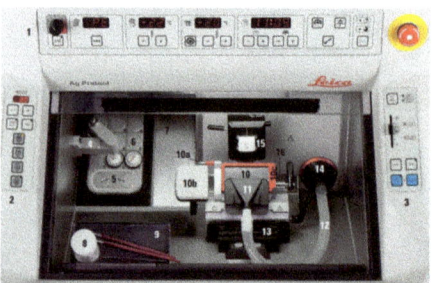

Fig. 6.32: Cryostat functional view—credits Leica team cryostat.

is must. After each use tissue debris from cryostat chamber must be cleared in biohazard bag. Debris can be picked using tissue paper or gauze piece soaked in 70% alcohol. It is important to minimize aerosols or spilling of debris in to open area.

Different disinfectant systems such as disinfectant spray, formaldehyde vapor, combination of disinfectant tray and UV light. These systems ensure a safe working environment, risk of infection by inhalation, and risk of contamination.

Cryostat support for producing good quality sections with following features:
- Vacuum, temperature and time control, lights, UV disinfection
- Electric cross feed
- Motorized sectioning
- Heat extractor
- Peltier element
- Freeze shelf, 15 positions
- Heat cold extractor, movable
- Shelf movable
- Blade holder

- Finger rest on blade holder
- Knife guard
- Extraction nozzle on the extraction hose
- Extraction hose for section waste
- Brush shelf
- Adapter piece for extraction hose
- Object head
- Waste tray

Method
- Tissue bit is placed on the disc/metal chuck and orient a mark on the disc/metal chuck helps to orient the specimen.
- Place the disc on **quick freezer shelf.** A heat extractor can be used to aid freezing and ensure good adherence and flat front block surface.
- Once the specimen is frozen insert the disc in the specimen head for sectioning
- Ensure before inserting disc/metal chuck in the specimen head
- Before mounting the specimen onto the microtome, ensure that the handwheel is in the locked position.
- A knife or blade is in place.
- Loosen clamping screw on the specimen head
- Insert the specimen disc/metal chuck in to opening of specimen head
- Tighten clamping screw
- Unlock the hand wheel
- Trim the specimen using coarse and precision feed buttons—use coarse feed button for moving specimen towards the cutting edge
- Set the section thickness to 6–10 µm using sections thickness knob

- ❖ Place the **anti roll guide plate** over the knife holder
  - Sections have a tendency to curl. Anti roll plate supports section to form flat sections.
  - Correct adjustment of anti-roll plate is very important to produce good sections.
  - It should be placed slightly above the knife edge.
- ❖ Cut serial sections by turning hand wheel with constant speed
- ❖ Pick up the sections and stained as desired.
- ❖ After completion of report, remove chuck out and submit frozen section bit for fixation and processing

End of day maintenance:
- ❖ Lock the hand wheel
- ❖ Remove frozen section waste with a brush
- ❖ Dispose waste as biohazard waste

Staining for Frozen Section

Rapid toludine blue—used as metachromatic stain
- ❖ Take a section on slide
- ❖ Stain in 1% toludine blue
- ❖ Wash in running tap water
- ❖ Mounting in glycerin

Rapid H&E stain:
- ❖ Take a section on slide
- ❖ Stain in Harri's hematoxylin for 2 minutes
- ❖ Differentiate in 0.5% acid alcohol quickly
- ❖ Blue in running tap water
- ❖ Stain in 1% eosin for 10 s
- ❖ Dehydrate, clear and mount in DPX

Quality control
To check frozen section accuracy, the tissue which is frozen is submitted for permanent preparation. This tissue is labeled as frozen section and processed separately from other additional tissue submitted for processing. If any diagnosis is differed in permanent section from frozen section diagnosis is notified immediately.

Troubles come across dealing frozen section
The consistency of frozen tissue block can be altered by varying tissue constituents and their ability to freeze. Optimize temperature according to tissue type. Reducing temperature will produce harder tissue block, raising the temperature makes tissue softer.
- **Freezing artifacts:** Result in holes in the sections. This is due to over cooling.
- Use of optimum temperature for freezing tissue is recommended
- Drying artifacts due to delay in fixation
- Ice crystals results in compressed sections
- **Sections curl over:** Adjust the antiroll plate
- **Sections getting washed off:** Apply adhesive to the slide before cutting

BIBLIOGRAPHY

1. Andrew Lisowski. Science of Tissue Processing. MS., HTL (ASCP). Leica Biosystems. https://www.leicabiosystems.com/us/knowledge-pathway
2. Bancroft's Theory and Practice of Histopathology Techniques, 5th edition.
3. Histological and Histochemical Methods, 4th edition.
4. Histotechnology Self-instructional Text, 4th edition

5. Microtomes and Microtome Knives—A Review and Proposed. Classification. Annal Dent Univ Malaya. 2012;19 (2).
6. Mounting Media—An Untouched Aspect. Oral Maxillofac Patho J. 2020;11(1): 20-24.
7. SR Peters. A Practical Guide to Frozen Section Technique. Springer.

STAINING TECHNIQUES

Introduction

Staining of tissue sections is last step in processing of sample preparation for microscopy. *Hematoxylin and Eosin (H&E)* is basic stain used routinely in for diagnosis in histopathology. This stain clearly differentiates nucleus, cytoplasm which allows identification of tissue components of type of epithelium, connective tissue, muscle, nervous tissue. Any stain other than H&E is referred as *Special Stain.* These stains are used if any additional information is required for diagnosis after viewing H&E stain. Special stains reveal structures like carbohydrates, mucins, reticulin fibers, basement membranes, also identify organisms such as bacteria, fungus, and pigments. The end result is stable, permanent which can be used using a light microscope.

Different dyes and chemicals are used for preparation of staining solutions. Use of appropriate acids, bases and buffers, quality of dyes is very important for preparation of stains and reagents, also some protocols even depend on process of oxidation and reduction.

For staining coupling jars are used in small laboratories, however, for large staining troughs or automation is frequently used in hospital laboratories/ corporate labs having volume of workload.

Basic Steps Involved in the Staining Protocol

This step is defined as ***Bring sections to water.***

- **Drying:** 3-4 μm thin sections are floated into water bath, then picked up and placed on a slide. The slides are then completely dried on a hot plate or in hot air oven to achieve adhesion. The temperature should be the same as melting point of the paraffin. Many automated stainers have drying ovens as part of the instrument so the time and temperature can be easily monitored. If oven/hot plate temperature is very high will result in cell distortion causing dark pyknotic nuclei or nuclear bubbling.
- **Deparaffinization:** Removal of paraffin wax from tissue sections—slides are placed in 2 changes of xylene for 5 minutes each.
- **Preparation for hydration:** Tissue sections are rehydrated, xylene is cleared. Slides are passed through 3 changes of alcohol for 5 minutes each (with alcohol strength decreasing with each sfollowing step).
- This step confirms the completion of rehydration process. Slides are placed in running tap water for 5 minutes—continue with desired staining protocol.
- **Post staining process:** Dehydration and clearing—slides are rapidly passed through 3 changes of alcohol followed by 2 changes of xylene. Clearing allows tissue sections to achieve refractive index with mounting medium.
- **Mounting, i.e., coverslipping:** When stain is complete, mounting is done by placing mounting medium DPX on coverslip and place the stained slide over it.

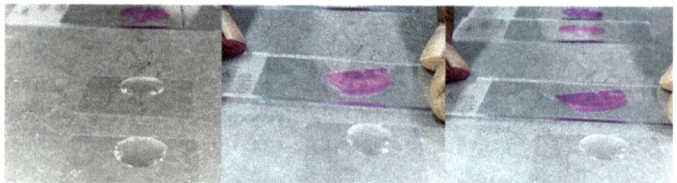

Fig. 6.33: Mounting of slide—manual method.

Mounting of Slides (Fig. 6.33)

- Bring sections to xylene.
- Arrange coverslips on blotting paper. Select appropriate size of coverslip.
- Add drop of mounting medium on coverslip.
- Place slide with stained section on the coverslip.
- Wipe edges of slides to remove xylene and excess of mounting medium.
- Arrange slides in a tray and submit slides for microscopy.

Automatic coverslipper is commercially **(Fig. 6.34)** available for larger workload. These are open systems for use of mounting medium. 400 slides are coverslipped in one hour. This allows user to select wet or dry choose between coverslipping. This is fully walk away system.

Mounting Medium

Mounting is also referred to as coverslipping.

Unmounted stained sections cannot be visualized under microscope. This is due to differences in refractive index of slide and tissue. Most of the tissues have refractive index 1.53 to 1.54 hence slides are mounted using transparent medium with similar

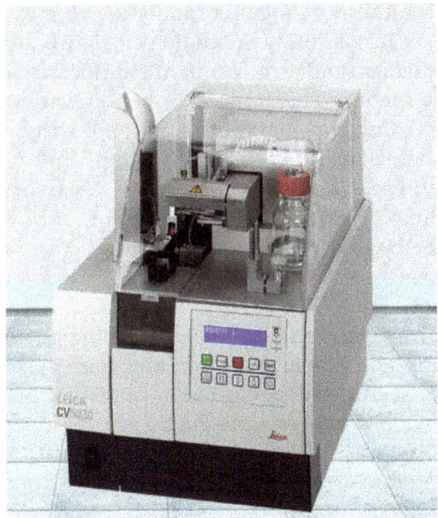

Fig. 6.34: Automatic coverslipper.

refractive index. Mounting of slides protect stained tissue sections from dust and damage during storage and make sections visible under microscope as well as enhance imaging quality. Mounting medium must be clear and transparent, easily miscible with xylene, nonreactive with stain and harden rapidly. Most of the laboratories now are using commercially available mounting medium.

Two types of mounting medium are available:
1. Aqueous mounting mediums are used with staining methods which alter on dehydration and clearing before mounting. Gelatin, gum arabic, syrup are three main components; Phenol,

thymol, sodium merthiolate are added as preservatives and are water based in nature. This mounting medium is not considered to be permanent and may dry up with the formation of bubbles on to the section. This process can be prevented by sealing coverslip using glue, nail polish, paraffin wax, varnish. The process of sealing is refferred as "ringing"

- *Glycerin jelly (refractive index 1.47)*—Used for fat stain

Gelatin	10 g
Distilled water	60 mL
Glycerin	70 mL
Phenol	0.25 mL

  Dissolve gelatin in distilled water using gentle heat. Add glycerin and phenol, mix well and store in screw capped bottle. Need to melt before use by keeping in hot water bath.

- *Apathy's medium (refractive index 1.52)*—Used for fluorescent microscopy.

Gum arabic	50 g
Cane sugar	50 g
Distilled water	50 mL
Thymol	0.05 g

  Dissolve and mix well, store in screw capped bottle.

- *Highman's modification of Apathy's medium (Refractive Index 1.52):* Recommended for use with metachromatic stain.

Gum Arabic	20 g
Cane sugar	20 g
Potassium acetate	20 g
Sodium merthiolate	10 mL
Distilled water	40 mL

  Dissolve and mix well, store in screw capped bottle.

- *Fructose syrup*-300 g/dL in distilled water (refractive index 1.47)—Used as a temporary mountant.

2. Resinous mounting medium; used for routinely processed tissue section slides using desired staining protocols such as H&E, special stains, immunohistochemistry. This is composed of resins and are in form of natural or synthetic are dissolved in xylene as solvent.

   Natural resinous medium –
   Canada balsam—refractive index 1.52–1.54
   Dammer balsam—refractive index 1.52–1.54
   Euparal—refractive index 1.48
   Kirkpatrik and Lendrum's DPX (refractive index 1.52) is routinely used mountant. This is synthetic resin made up of,

Distrene 80	10 g
Dibutylphthalate	5 mL
Xylene	35 mL

   However, in routine commercially available mountant DPX (Distyrene Plasticizer xylene) is used.

Concept of Staining

In histology, stains are coloured compounds that allows visualizing of cells and tissue components under the light microscope. The end result is stable and permanent. Staining is usually done on tissue sections and cell smears. Use of quality dyes, appropriate acids, bases, and buffers are part of successful staining process. Stain uptake is due to affinity between dye and tissue or reagent and tissue. Tissues are referred to as acidophilic and basophilic on the basis of their affinity with stains. Factors contributing to this affinity are electrostatic bond, van der Waals forces, hydrogen bonding, hydrophobic interaction, covalent bonding.

Classification of Dyes

- Natural dyes—carmine, saffron, hematoxylin, indigo, alizarin red, berry, vegetable juices and many more.
- Saffron was applied on sections of muscle fiber by Antonie van Leeuwenhoek in 1714.
- Carmine derived from insect dactylopius coccus used by Joseph Gerlach in 1858
- Hematoxylin is a natural dye used in routine; used by Wilhelm Waldeyer in 1863

Synthetic Dyes

The first synthetic dyes aniline dye was accidently evolved in 1856 by William Perkin. Later in 1900, 47 different dye structures of aniline were factory made and this led to development of various histochemical stains.

Most of the dyes are synthesized from benzene and its derivative.

Dye

Dye is a coloured compound that chemically binds with the tissue component to give stable colored end product.

Formation of Dye

All dyes are aromatic benzene ring compound (C_6H_6) that possess the twin properties, to color and ability to bind tissue. Basically, the benzene ring compound is colorless by itself. Chromogen and Auxo chrome are attached to benzene ring to form dye complex.

Quinoid structure chromophore

Quinoid rings are found in many dyes. Hematoxylin on oxidization gets quinoid arrangement in lieu of two hydrogen atoms and used as active nuclear stain.

Chromogen

Chromogen is the substance possessing chromophore group. Chromophore is the arrangement of atoms within chromogen that is responsible for absorption of light in the visible part of spectrum. Usually, they are represented as nitrogen, carbon, oxygen, and sulfur that have alternate single and double bonds.

Classification of dyes by chromophoric group		
Chromophore group		*Dyes*
Nitro group	—NO$_2$	Picric acid, martius yellow
Nitroso group	—N==O	Naphthol green Y, naphthol green B
Azo group	—N==N	Orange G, biebrich scarlet, bismarck brown, alcian yellow, Sudan IV, oil red O, Sudan Black B, Congo Red, ponceau xylidine, chromotrope 2R,
Thiazine dyes	—C==S	Toluidine blue, Methylene blue, Azure A
Arylmethane dyes	==N or O	Aniline blue, light green, fast green FCF, basic fuchsin, acid fuchsin, malachite green, pararosaniline, aniline blue
Thiazole group	—C==N	Hematoxylin
Xanthene dyes	==N R'R",==O Several subgroups	Eosin, phloxine, rhodamine B
Phthalocyanine		Alcian blue 8GX, luxel fast blue
Azine/oxazine dyes	C—O==C C—N==C	Cresyl violet, orcein, neutral red
Anthraquinone dyes		Carminic acid, Alizarin red, nuclear fast red

Auxochrome

The word is derived from two roots. The prefix auxo is from auxein and means increased. The second part, chrome means color, so the basic meaning of auxochrome is color increaser (Wikipedia).

The auxochrome which is side chain attached to chromogen may be (1) an ionizable group (2) a group that reacts to form covalent bond with a substrate (3) an arrangement of atoms that forms coordinate bonds with metal ions (mordants).

Example of auxochrome groups—hydroxyl (—OH), carboxyl (—COOH), sulfonic group (—HSO_4) are responsible for acid ionization; amino (—NH_2) for basic ionization and other basic groups such as —N==N,—N.

A fluorochrome absorbs ultraviolet, violet, blue or green light and emits light of longer wavelength. This is used in fluorescent microscopy.

Action for Dye Binding

Reagent Tissue Interaction

Coulombic attractions have been termed salt links or electrostatic bonds.

- **Ionic binding:** Linkage formed from electrostatic attraction between oppositely charged ions in tissue—stain interaction. Negative (anionic) dye which is acidic combines positively charged tissue components. Salts are added to increase intensity of staining reaction hence, also considered as salt linkage.
- **Hydrogen bonding:** This bonding arises when hydrogen atoms lie between two electronegative atoms like oxygen, nitrogen. For example, water (H_2O) is a good solvent; readily forms hydrogen bonds with the solute.

- **Van der Waals force:** These are weak forces and can act only between two molecules that are already close together. This involves different intermolecular attractions—dipole-dipole, dipole induced dispersion forces. They are effective over a short distance. For example, adhesion of the section to the slide involves Van der Waals reaction between section and slide.
- **Covalent bonding:** This bonding involves sharing electrons. This can occur between stain and the tissue. They form very strong bonds and are not easily broken. For example, mordant lake formation.

Solvent-Solvent Interaction

Hydrophobic binding: These bindings are responsible for penetration of oil soluble dyes into lipids and for their retention at hydrophobic binding sites in the tissue.

Stain—Stain Interaction

Dye aggregation: Dye molecules attract each other forming dye aggregates. For example, metachromatic staining using toluidine blue stain.

Classification of Dyes by their Action

- **Basic dyes:** Basic dyes are cationic which are attached by electrostatic forces to anions. Basophilic is the term used for components of a cell tissue which take up basic stain. Nuclei are basophilic.
- **Acid dyes:** Acid dyes are anionic. They form salts with the ionized amino groups of proteins particularly cationic groups in cells and tissues. Acidophilic is the term applied to group which shows affinity to acid dyes. The cytoplasm is usually acidophilic.

- ❖ **Neutral dyes:** These are a mixture of acid and basic dyes, for example, Romanowsky stains which will stain both nucleus and cytoplasm.
- ❖ **Mordant dyes:** A mordant is a polyvalent metal which forms a link between tissue and dye. Aluminium and ferric ions are two commonly used metal salts. The dye and mordant are attached with each other by means of chelation—covalent and this coordinate bond are referred as LAKE.
  - Mordant and dyes can be combined in three ways,
  - *Onchrome:* Mordant is used first followed by dye; for example, iron hematoxylin
  - *Metachrome:* Mordant and dyes are mixed and used; for example, alum haematoxylin
- ❖ **Solvent dyes:** Dyes that do not dissolve in water are soluble in only hydrophobic solvents; fat stain.
- ❖ **Adsorption:** This is defined as adhesion of molecules together and are loosely held by the surface. This is a physical reaction dependent on the charge of dye and material to be stained. For example, eosin is adsorbed by tissue section followed by action of 95% alcohol with differentiation of eosin stain and quick dehydration process. If slides are left for longer time in 95% alcohol will remove eosin resulting in weak stain.
- ❖ **Metachromatic dye:** The dye that stains in different color. Color change is commonly observed from blue to violet or yellow to orange. Color absorption at different wavelengths is due to dye-to-dye interaction.
- ❖ **Argyrophil:** Affinity for silver salts which are subsequently reduced to black metallic silver.
- ❖ **Argentaffin:** Affinity for silver salts and are capable of reducing to black metallic silver without the need of a reducing agent.
- ❖ **Counter stain:** The term used with many staining methods, stating that counter stain with, for example light green and many more.

This second dye to accentuate the primary dye without interfering with the primary dye.

Dye Selection

Purchase of dye certified by Biological Stain Commission is recommended as dye impurities have shown effects on staining. Altered staining intensity is observed. Impurities may change staining pattern by altering the nature and mechanisms of such effects depending on the type of impurity, the staining procedure and tissue substrate.

Guidelines to Avoid Problems in Staining

- Use chemically clean glassware of appropriate type and size to prepare stain and reagents.
- Label all stains and reagents clearly.
- Use graded stains and reagents.
- Keep check on storage conditions, for example, light proof (dark) bottle or refrigeration.
- Standardize staining protocol.
- Prepare control database for validation of staining protocol.
- Daily control run is must.
- Unexpected stain reaction—pH of stain alters the reaction.
- Choose fixative as recommended in staining protocol.

Hematoxylin and Eosin Stain

Routinely used staining protocol in all histopathology laboratories word wide.

Hematoxylin

Hematoxylin is extracted from the logwood of the tree Haematoxylum campechianum. It is important to realize that Hematoxylin itself is not a stain; it is an oxidation product hematin which is the natural dye.

Hematin can be produced from Hematoxylin in two forms:
1. **Natural oxidation:** Dyes can be oxidized by exposure to light and air. The process is also referred as "Ripening". A slow process, can even take 3–4 months for ripening but solutions will have long shelf life. For example, Ehrlich's and Delafield's hematoxylin.
2. **Chemical oxidation:** Using sodium iodate–Mayer's Haematoxylin, or mercuric oxide—Harri's hematoxylin.

This dye can be used immediately upon preparation. The oxidation process is rapid but the solution does not have a long shelf life. Hence it is recommended to prepare stock sufficient for one month.

Haematin is anionic and has poor affinity for tissue. The use of mordant/metal complex in combination with hematin allows it to combined with tissue. It binds to anionic tissue sites such as nuclear chromatin. Thus, hematoxylin is one of the best nuclear stains used in different staining methods.

Eosin

Eosin, xanthene dye is also a salt that dissociates in water into ions. Its negative ion, which is acidic in nature, readily combines with positively charged regions of cellular macromolecules, especially positively charged regions of cytoplasmic proteins, coloring them a variety of hues, ranging from pink to red to orange.

Any substance, cell, or tissue, that tends to be stained in this way by eosin is said to be acidophilic or eosinophilic. Eosinophilic components are cationic compounds that have an affinity for that acid dye.

Eosin-Phloxine solution will produce a cytoplasmic stain where muscle is clearly differentiated from collagen and red cells stain bright red.

1% Phloxine B	10 mL
1% Eosin Y	100 mL
95% alcohol	780 mL
Glacial acetic acid	4 mL

1% Eosin

Eosin Y	4 g
Distilled water	80 mL
Absolute alcohol	320 mL
Glacial acetic acid	0.4 mL

Note: Alcoholic preparation of eosin gives sharp staining contrast

Progressive and Regressive Staining, Differentiation, Bluing

- Progressive staining is a direct staining method. The tissue section is allowed to be in staining solution until desired uptake of color is achieved.
- Regressive staining is an indirect staining method. Tissue sections are over stained. Excess of stain is removed using differentiation step to achieve desired staining reaction. This breaks covalent bonds and removes just excess of hematoxylin.
- **Differentiation:** Process of removal of excess stain. Differentiation acts on the mordant dye linkages.
  Acid alcohol—Differentiating solution.
  Add 1 mL of concentrated hydrochloric acid is added to 70% alcohol.
- **Bluing:** Alum haematoxylin is used regressively. Sections are differentiated using acid alcohol followed by bluing by placing slides in running tap water. Alum basically acidic in nature tend to dissociate in water by forming free hydroxyl group results in

bluing. This process reforms mordant dye linkages. Washing in running tap water is used for bluing in routine however alkaline solutions more than pH 8.0 such as Scott's water, lithium carbonate solution. Bluing is pH dependent reaction.

Bluing Solutions

- **Alcoholic ammonia solution:** Add 1–2 drops of ammonia solution in 100 mL of 70% alcohol.
- **Lithium carbonate solution:** 1 g of lithium carbonate in 100 mL of distilled water.
- **Scott's tap water (SWTS)**

  Magnesium sulfate   10 g
  Sodium carbonate   2 g
  Distilled water   1000 mL

  Mix well. To be changed after each batch of staining.

Note: Bluing is a very important step and never be rushed. This will result in the fading of slides in few weeks.

Preparation of Hematoxylin Stains

Haematoxylin solutions are classified according to the use of mordants.

Type of Hematoxylin	Mordants used
Alum hematoxylin	Aluminium in form of potassium alum or aluminium alum
Iron hematoxylin	Using Iron salts—ferric chloride, ferric ammonium sulfate
Lead hematoxylin	Lead salts
Tungsten hematoxylin	Phosphotungstic acid
Molybdenum hematoxylin	Molybdic acid

Iron Hematoxylin

Weigert's Iron Hematoxylin

This belongs to the iron hematoxylin group. Ferric chloride is used is mordant/oxidant.

Due to over oxidation of hematoxylin ferric chloride and hematoxylin solutions are prepared and stored separately. Ferric chloride is also used as differentiating fluid after hematoxylin staining.

Weigert's iron hematoxylin is used as nuclear in trichrome methods. When stained using alum hematoxylin nuclear staining fades when due to use of acidic stains in subsequent staining steps in trichrome stains.

Reagents

Stock Solution

1. Hematoxyline   1 g m
    95% alcohol   100 mL
2. 29% Ferric chloride   4 mL
    Conc. hydrochloric acid   1 mL
    Distilled water   100 mL

Working Solution

Mix equal parts of 1 and 2 just before use. The mixture should be violet blue and must be discarded if it is brown.

Alum Hematoxylin

❖ **Mayer's hematoxylin (1901)**
  Potassium or ammonium alum   50 g
  Hematoxylin   1 g

Sodium iodate	0.2 g
Citric acid	1g
Chloral hydrate	50 g
Distilled water	1,000 mL

Dissolve the above contents in given order in 750 mL warm distilled water. Magnetic stirrer can accelerate the mixing of reagents. Chloral hydrate acts as a preservative. Citric acid enhances the staining reaction.

❖ **Harri's hematoxylin (1900)**

Hematoxylin	5 g
Ethyl alcohol	50 mL
Potassium or ammonium alum	100 g
Distilled water	950 mL
Mercuric oxide	2.5 g
Glacial acetic acid	40 mL

Dissolve hematoxylin in alcohol. Dissolve alum in water by aid of heat. Remove from heat and mix the two solutions. Heat the mixture to boiling point. Remove from heat and add mercuric oxide. As soon as mixture turns a dark purple, cool quickly by plunging the vessel into cold water. When cool, add 40 mL of glacial acetic acid to enhance nuclear stain.

Note: Acetic acid enhances staining of nuclei however if added in whole hematoxyline will lead to shorter shelf life of the stain. It is better to be used in working solution.

❖ **Delafield's hematoxylin (1885)**

Hematoxylin	4 g
95% Ethanol	125 mL
Saturated ammonium Alum (15 g/100 mL)	400 mL
Glycerin	100 mL

Hematoxylin is dissolved in 25 mL of ethanol, which is warmed in the water bath. Then added to alum solution and allowed to stand in air and light for 5–7 days. Filter the solution. Add Glycerin and the remaining 100 mL 95% ethanol. This solution is allowed to ripen naturally in air and light for 3 months. Filter and use.

❖ **Ehrlich's Hematoxylin (1886)**

Hematoxylin	2 g
Absolute alcohol	100 mL
Glycerin	100 mL
Glacial acetic acid	10 mL
Potassium Alum	15 g

Haematoxylin is dissolved in absolute alcohol. Add glacial acetic acid and glycerin. Dissolve alum in the distilled water with the help of heat and shaking. Once alum is dissolved cool the solution. Then add hematoxylin, glycerin, glacial acetic acid mixture to alum. Mix well. Allow it to ripen naturally. It may take 8 weeks.

This hematoxylin can be artificially ripened by adding 0.2 g sodium iodate.

Glycerin stabilizes solution and prevents over oxidation of hematoxylin.

This is stable hematoxylin if ripened naturally.

❖ **Gill's hematoxylin (1974)**

Hematoxylin	2 g
Sodium iodate	0.2 g
Aluminum sulfate	17.6 g
Distilled water	750 mL
Ethylene glycol	250 mL
Glacial acetic acid	20 mL

Ethylene glycol is mixed with distilled water and hematoxylin is added and dissolved. Sodium iodate (as oxidizer) is added, and then aluminum sulfate is added. Finally glacial acetic acid is added and stirred using magnetic stirrer. The stain is ready for use. Allow it to ripen at 37°C for one week.

- **Celestine blue–alum hematoxylin method**

This method utilizes combination of celestine blue, ferric alum with alum hematoxyline. Celestin blue is resistant to the effects of acid and along with ferric alum (mordant) strengthen bond between nucleus and alum hematoxyline. Celestine blue hemalum is used as a nuclear stain in Martius Scarlet Blue method for fibrin.

Reagents

Celestin blue	2.5 g
Ferric ammonium sulfate	25 g
Glycerin	70 mL
Distilled water	500 mL

Dissolve ferric ammonium sulfate in distilled water with stirring. Mix well.

Add celestin blue to the mixture; the mixture is then boiled for few minutes. After cooling filter, the stain and add glycerin. Filter before use.

Method

- Deparaffinize sections and hydrate through graded alcohols to water
- Stain in celestin blue for 5 minutes
- Stain in alum hematoxylin (e.g., Mayer's) for 5 minutes
- Wash in water until blue
- Proceed with required staining technique.

Manual H&E Staining Protocol

- **Deparaffinization**
  Xylene I   5 minutes
  Xylene II   5 minutes
- **Rehydration**
  Isopropyl alcohol I   5 minutes
  Isopropyl alcohol II   5 minutes
- Running tap water
- *Harri's hematoxylin*   5–7 minutes
- Running tap water
- *Differentiate* in 1% acid alcohol
- Bluing – Running tap water   10 minutes
- Eosin   30 seconds
- **Dehydration**
  - Isopropyl alcohol I   10 seconds
  - Isopropyl alcohol II   10 seconds
  - Isopropyl alcohol III 10 seconds
- **Clearing**
  Xylene I   5 minutes
  Xylene II   5 minutes
  Blot dry to clean the slide.
  Mount in DPX.
  Results—(Figs. 6.35A and B)
  Nuclei—Blue
  Muscle, keratin, coarse elastic, fibrin—red
  Collagen, reticulin, amyloid—pink

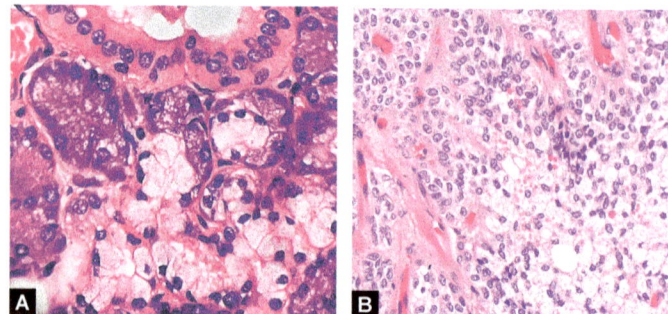

Figs. 6.35A and B: H&E stained slides.

hallmark of Ideal Processing

- Excellent morphological presentation of tissue
- Nuclei with various crisp chromatin pattern and crisp blue nuclear membrane
- Cytoplasm stained well with different intensities of eosin.

Automation for H&E Staining (Figs. 6.36A to C)

Automated platforms are now available for hematoxylin eosin stain. Different kinds of stainers is in practice; automation with the large work load has eased work of technical staff but training for understanding mechanism of instrument is mandatory for working. Progressive staining protocol is recommended. Haematoxylin eosin, PAP stain, special stains can be performed on automation.

Types of automation
1. **Circular type:** Carousel type mechanism (Shandon)
    - Touch control panel enabling different programs.

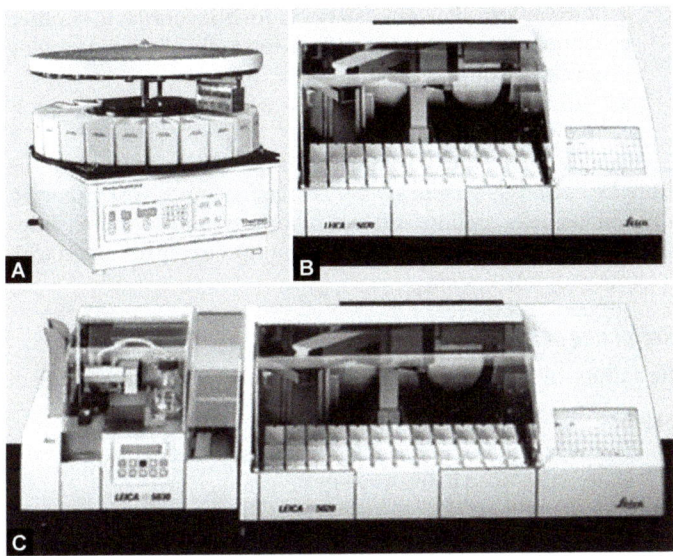

Figs. 6.36A to C: Automation for H&E staining.

- Equipment has a water wash facility which enables water to enter in the trough (dishes) through an inlet on to lower outside wall. The outlet is a weir at the rear of the trough. This weir controls the level of water in the trough and directs excess water into a circular water collection.
2. **Linear type:** Robotic arm is used to transfer the slides from one jar to another (Leica)
    - Touch control panel enabling different programs.
    - Linear type machines have the advantage of continuous loading and unloading of slides.

- Robotic arm allows transfer of slides from one jar to another.
- Optional oven modules with up to 4 racks allow slide drying and dewaxing.
- Multiple-valve design activates water flow only when it is really needed.

Integrated system of stainer and coverslipper is available from Leica. In this system stainer and coverslipper are connected through transfer station. A novel robotic system transfers slides from staining in to coverslipper. The equipment is designed with trouble shooting system.

Restaining of HE Slides

Restaining of slides is usually done whenever stained slide is faded.

Method
- The coverslip from previously stained slides is removed.
- Slides are placed in fresh xylene.
- Slides are rinsed in fresh xylene after the cover slip is removed.
- Slides are then passed through two changes of absolute alcohol.
- Slides are decolorized in 1% acid alcohol until section is colorless.
- Slides are washed thoroughly in running tap water for 10–15 minutes.
- Then the slides are stained as routine H&E procedure.

Rapid restaining of HE slides: After removing coverslip slide is to be cleared by placing in xylene and alcohol. Rinse in running tap water. Place in 1% ammonia in 70% of alcohol (freshly prepared) for 2–3 minutes or till cytoplasmic stain is dissolved. Rinse in tap water for 1–2 minutes. Counterstain with eosin for 30 seconds. Dehydrate, clear and mount.

Quality Control

- Refer to operator's manual for cleaning and maintenance of the autostainer.
- Daily filter the hematoxylin with Whatman filter paper no. 1
- Daily check levels of stains and reagents.
- Maintain log of change of stains and reagents

Trouble Shooting—H&E Stain

Efficacy of the hematoxylin can be checked by adding a few drops of hematoxylin solution to tap water. It has to convert blue to purple color immediately.

If it changes color slowly or turns red brown hematoxylin is not to be used. It is oxidized in excess.

Problems in H&E result in:
- **Patchy staining can be due to less deparaffinization:** Slides will have to be destained and stained again.
- **Hazy sections can result because of less dehydration:** Repeat dehydration with fresh change of alcohol.
  - Xylene and alcohol have to be replaced regularly. Change of reagent log must be maintained.
- **Differentiation:** Over differentiation will be cause of faint nuclear staining.
  - Restain with hematoxylin
  - Less differentiation will give very dark staining of hematoxylin and eosin with no contrast. Prepare fresh differentiating solution.
- **Pale or no nuclear staining:** Repeat staining with fresh haematoxylin.

❖ **Nuclei not crisp, "Smudgy" nuclei, nuclear bubbling or no distinct chromatin pattern:** Poor or incomplete fixation, incomplete dehydration, slides were exposed to excess heat during processing or drying.

BIBLIOGRAPHY

1. Lillie and Fullmer NM. Histopathologic technic and practical histochemistry. 1976, Fourth edition.
2. K Lakshminarayan. Histological techniques.
3. Bancroft JD and Stevens A. Theory and practice of histological techniques, 5th edition.
4. John A Kiernan. Classification and naming of dyes, stains and fluorochromes.
5. Freida L Carson. Histotechnology: A Self Instructional Text, 4th edition.

CHAPTER 7

Immunohistochemistry

INTRODUCTION

The immunohistochemistry is the technique used to detect antigens in the tissue sections or cell smears based on the antigen antibody recognition with the help of a labeling system which allows to visualize reproducible results for light microscopy. Experts have referred this powerful technique as "Brown revolution" Over last more than four decades, the number of tests in immunohistochemistry are increased and currently departments associated with cancer hospitals/corporate laboratories are using more than 130 markers for the same.

Immunohistochemistry has evolved as an important and commonly used test in histopathology and plays an important role in identifying tumors for diagnosis and classification, prognosis, and treatment for cancer. The sensitivity of the technique has improved over a period of years from immunofluorescence labeled antibody system to labeled polymer based systems and development of monoclonal antibodies. Immunohistochemistry can be performed on routinely formalin fixed paraffin embedded (FFPE) tissue sections, frozen sections, and cytology preparation. Slides can always be reviewed as the end result with chromogen substate is permanent.

Effects of tissue fixation is greatly improved with the help of heat induced antigen retrieval methods in early 1990. The advantage of the use of FFPE that antigen expression can be seen in archival material and be useful for research purposes.

Introduction of companion diagnostic terminology in immunohistochemistry wherein test results are directly associated with targeted therapy for patients. Companion diagnostic test belongs to category class III medical device by FDA. Her-2-neu testing was approved by FDA in 1998 and lately PDL1. This concept of companion diagnostic test has led stringent monitoring of test performances, especially for reproducibility of results hence standardization of immunohistochemistry protocol is very important.

The introduction of automation in immunostaining was of great help to manage test volumes, report turnaround time and test standardization.

Technical Developments

- **Coons, Creech, Jones 1941:** Immunofluorescence technique. (FITC conjugate), first developed an immunofluorescence technique to detect corresponding antigens in frozen tissue sections. Antibody was labeled with fluorescent dye (Fluorescein isocyanate). Based on the principle of the immunofluorescence technique new labels, alternate labeling techniques were identified. However, IFA techniques had its own limitations i.e., fading of slides, hard to get permanent preparation, lack of morphologic details and need of fluorescent microscope.
- **Nakane and Pierce 1966:** Development of enzyme horseradish peroxidase allowed visualization of the labeled antibody by light microscopy in the presence of a suitable colorogenic substrate system such as diaminobenzidine (DAB).

- **Sternberger et al. 1979:** Unlabeled antibody method (peroxidase anti peroxidase-PAP technique). First three step sandwich method—primary antibody + secondary antibody + PAP immune complex. APAAP—alkaline phosphatase anti alkaline phosphatase technique using same principle was first developed by Cordell et al. in 1984.
- **Kohler and Milstein, 1975:** Received Nobel prize for the development of hybridoma techniques; Revolution in IHC—production of monoclonal antibodies.
- **Huang, 1975:** Enzyme digestion for the recovery retrieval (introduced antigen trypsin)
- **Hsu and collegues,1981:** Avidin—biotin, another unlabeled method, more sensitive Cordell et al. 1984—APAAP technique.
- **Bobrow and colleagues 1989:** Catalyzed reporter deposition techniques: were further adapted to IHC (Tyramine amplification)
- **Pluzek 1993:** New direct technique first reported in 1993 Pluzek et al. This technique involves dextran polymer backbone to which multiple antibodies and enzyme molecules are conjugated by increasing sensitivity in comparison of traditional techniques.
- **Shi et al. 1991:** Heat pretreatment for antigen retrieval (use of heavy metals), Cattoretti et al. 1993—heat pretreatment (pH 6.0 citrate buffer, safe); Norton 1994—use of pressure cooker for antigen retrieval. Later several modifications antigen retrieval methods and incubation timings were studied to overcome formalin fixation effect.
- **Automation:** In the 1980s David Brigati developed the first automated immunostainer reagent application on slides and washing between the steps was made possible using a capillary action. In today's era different semiautomated and

fully-automated immunostainer platforms are available for use in the laboratory.
- **Spieker-Polet 1995:** Production of rabbit monoclonal antibodies.

Antigen Antibody Reaction

Identification of specific tissue components (antigen) is feasible by means of antigen/antibody reaction. The reaction is based on affinity between antigen and antibody. This highly precise and specific binding is compared with lock (antibody) and key (antigen) mechanism.

Affinity

Affinity is the strength of binding i.e., measures the strength of interaction between an epitope and an antibody's binding site. They bind through a combination of different mechanisms like hydrogen bonds, electrostatic forces, and van der Waals force to form stable immune complex. B lymphocytes, T lymphocytes, macrophages are major components in immune system.

Antigen

An antigen is a substance which can stimulate production of antibodies resulting in immune response and bears one or more antibody binding sites. The site at which antigen antibody reacts is antigenic determinant or epitope. Epitopes are small parts of antigens that generate a specific antibody during response. These are group of 5 to 8 amino acids or monosaccharide units and represent only a small part of an antigen (peptides, amino acids, polysaccharides, lipids, and nucleic acids when combined with amino acid and polysaccharide) units which bind specifically to an antibody. Antigen antibody recognition is based on the three-dimensional structure of protein or some other antigen which may be compromised due to formalin fixation, i.e., altering or masking of protein component. This can be restored using antigen retrieval (AR) protocols.

Antibody

An antibody is a protein molecule which forms immune complex in presence of another molecule antigen. It is produced by B cells. These activated B cells are transformed into plasma cells that binds to specific antigen. This is referred to as humoral response.

There are five types of antibodies IgG, IgM, IgA, IgD and IgE.

Basic monomer unit of antibody **(Fig. 7.1)** consists—two identical light chains and two identical heavy chains joined to form a "Y" shaped molecule. The light chains are either a kappa or a lambda pair and heavy chains comprise gamma, alpha, mu, delta, and epsilon. These are connected together by disulfide (S—S) bonds and noncovalent bonds. "Y" molecule of antibody is composed of Fab variable fragment and constant Fc end. Variable fragments at the terminal ends of "Y" arm are responsible for the active site formation in the antibodies.

Antibodies are generated by immunizing (injecting) animals with purified antigen. The animal responds by producing antibodies that specifically recognize and bind to the antigen.

The majority of antibodies used in immunohistochemistry are IgG. Specificity and sensitivity are two specific criteria used for selection of antibody in immunohistochemistry.

The antibodies used for specific detection can be polyclonal or monoclonal.

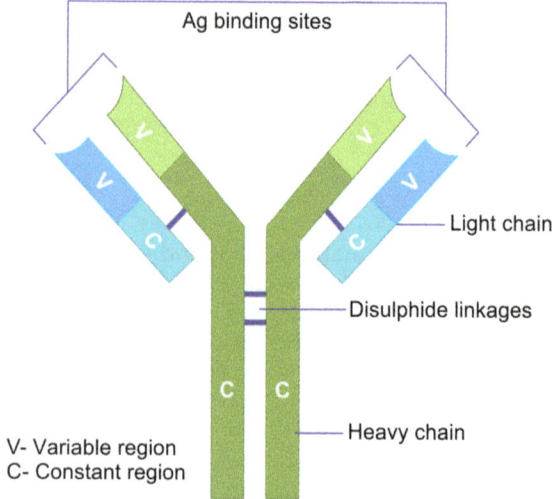

Fig. 7.1: Structure of antibody.

The main difference between monoclonal and polyclonal antibodies is that monoclonal antibodies are produced by the same clone of plasma B cells, and they bind to a unique epitope whereas polyclonal antibodies are produced by different clones of plasma B cells, and they bind to the different epitopes in the same antigen.

Polyclonal Antibodies

Heterogeneous population of antibodies against several epitopes hence referred as polyclonal (**Fig. 7.2**).

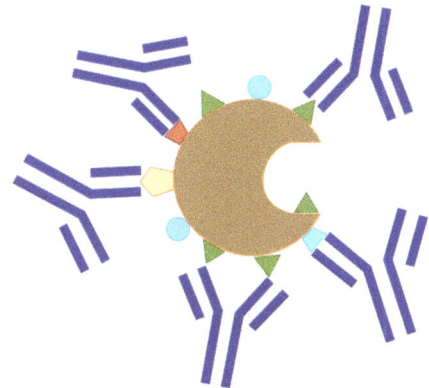

Fig. 7.2: Polyclonal antibody.

Rabbit is the most commonly used animal for production of polyclonal antibodies. Each type of antibodies in the mixture are originated from a specific clone of plasma B cells. Thereby, the production of polyclonal antibodies employs multiple clones of plasma B cells. The animal is immunized with an immunogen bearing antigen of interest. Immunization is performed subcutaneously. Blood is collected from the ear of the rabbit. Serum is separated from blood by centrifugation and is further purified for production of antibodies. Purification is done by means of either protein purification or antigen affinity chromatography. Purified antibodies are heterogeneous mixture of antibodies react with various epitopes on an antigen likely to exhibit batch to batch variation.

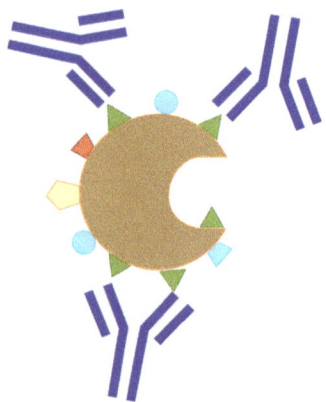

Fig. 7.3: Monoclonal antibodies.

Polyclonal antibody is highly sensitive because it binds to multiple epitopes but this also means it is not selective resulting in nonspecific staining. Titers used to stain tissue must be carefully selected to ensure no false positive staining.

Monoclonal Antibodies

Homogenous population of monoclonal antibodies (**Fig. 7.3**) against a single epitope.

Kohler and Milstein received the Nobel prize for the development of hybridoma techniques. This is revolutionary step in the field of immunohistochemistry. They introduced a wide range of highly specific monoclonal of antibodies.

Monoclonal antibodies (**Fig. 7.4**) are made by fusing myeloma cells with spleen cells from mouse that has been immunized with

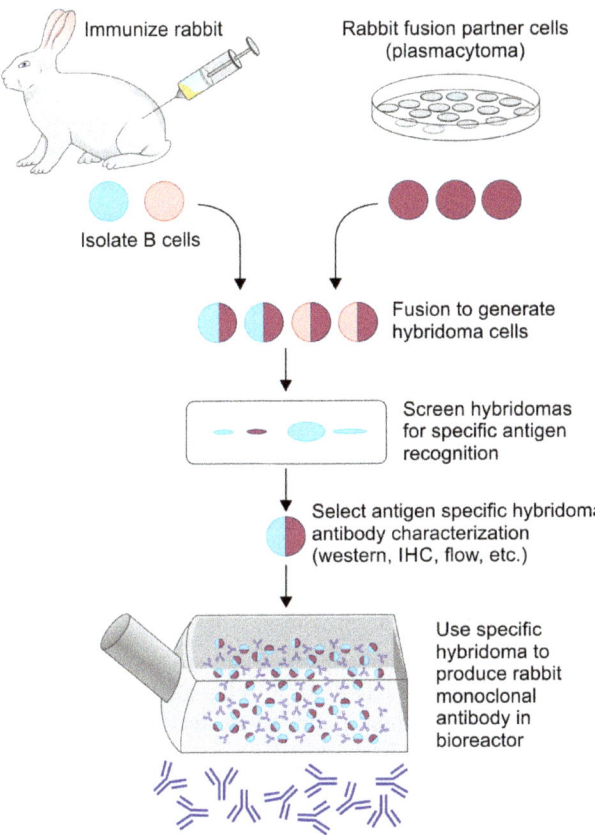

Fig. 7.4: Production of monoclonal antibodies.

desired antigen. Monoclonal antibodies are raised in tissue culture media (culture supernatant) or generated from hybridoma cells injected in peritoneal cavity (ascitic fluid). These are immortalized by fusion with hybridoma cells, allowing for long-term generation of identical monoclonal antibodies. Monoclonal antibodies were mostly from mice because of a strong myeloma cell line until latest devolvement of rabbit monoclonal. Rabbit myeloma cell line has higher fusion efficiency and makes the stable hybridoma achievable for obtaining rabbit monoclonals.

Monoclonal antibodies can be characterized, standardized and produced in unlimited quantities. The advantages of monoclonal antibodies include high homogeneity, the absence of nonspecific antibodies, no batch-to-batch variation.

Labeling Methods

Immunohistochemistry is a technique of visualizing tissue antigen using different labels and labeling methods. Over the period of years sensitivity of technique has improved from single layer labeling to polymer-based technique. Development of different techniques has enabled visualization of antigen antibody reaction using different types of specimen preparation. Different Labels are used to determine intensification to improve sensitivity of technique.

There are different labeling methods are available to identify tissue antigens. Broadly methods are classified as:
- Direct method in which a label is attached to the antibody which reacts directly with tissue antigen.
- Indirect method in which an unlabeled antibody is employed as an antigen for a labeled secondary antibody.

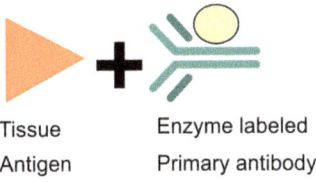

Fig. 7.5: Direct labeling method.

Direct Method (Fig. 7.5)

Tissue + Enzyme labeled primary antibody:
The simplest short and quick method, but had limitations.

In this one step staining method primary antibody is tagged with enzyme label which binds directly to antigen being stained for. The antibody may be labeled with FITC or other fluorescent dyes is visualized with fluorescence microscope or labeled with enzyme such as horse radish peroxidase (HRP), alkaline phosphatase, glucose oxidase followed by counterstained with chromogen and visualized using light microscope. Application of direct techniques is mainly used for kidney biopsies and skin lesions. However, due to lack of sensitivity the technique has limitations in tumor diagnosis.

Two Step Indirect Method (Fig. 7.6)

Tissue + Primary antibody + Enzyme labeled secondary antibody
This method involves unconjugated primary antibody is allowed to bind to antigen being stained for with the help of enzyme labeled secondary antibody and visualized using chromogen substrate of choice. If labeled with fluorescent dye is called as indirect immunofluorescence method. This modification in technique has improved sensitivity of method. Secondary antibody must be of same species as primary antibody applied in this method.

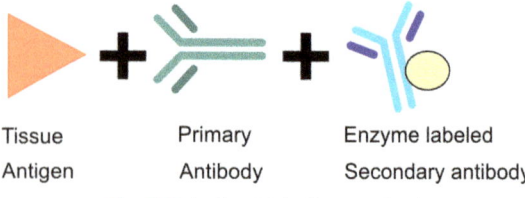

Fig. 7.6: Indirect labeling method.

Three Step Indirect Method

The three-step method (enzyme bridge method) wherein stable complex is formed using primary antibody, link antibody (secondary unlabeled), enzyme anti enzyme complex such as peroxidase anti peroxidase (PAP) or alkaline phosphatase anti alkaline phosphatase (APAAP).

Peroxidase Anti Peroxidase Method—PAP (Fig. 7.7)

Tissue + Primary antibody + link antibody (Secondary unlabeled) + HRP visualized using chromogen substrate (DAB).

The enzyme used is horseradish peroxidase (HRP) which is conjugated with the antibody of same species as primary antibody via link antibody.

Alkaline Phosphatase Anti Alkaline Phosphatase—APAAP (Fig. 7.8)

Tissue + Primary antibody + link antibody (Secondary unlabeled) + ALP visualized using chromogen substrate.

Enzyme alkaline phosphatase acts on naphthol-as-phosphate as substrate. This couples with diazonium salts. This technique is mostly used with bone marrow and peripheral smears.

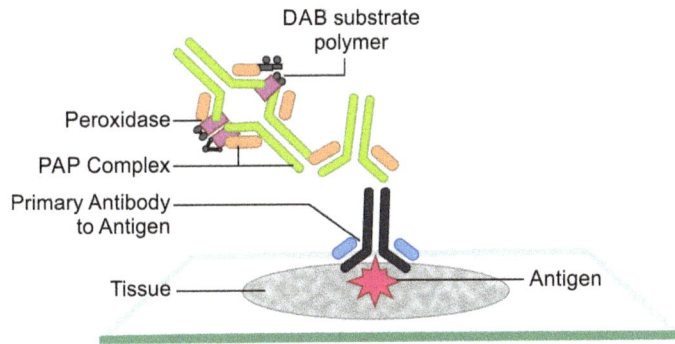

Fig. 7.7: PAP method.

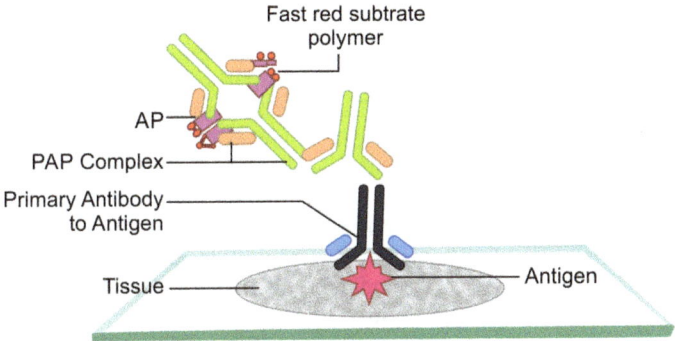

Fig. 7.8: APAAP method.

Avidin Biotin Methods—(Fig. 7.9)

This technique is based on high affinity of avidin for biotin. Avidin is a large glycoprotein possessing four high affinity binding sites

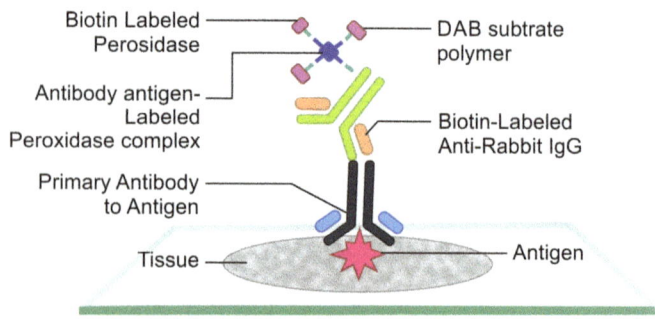

Fig. 7.9: ABC method (detection system).

for biotin a small vitamin molecule. Modification of avidin biotin method is replacement of avidin with streptavidin which can be isolated from bacillus Streptomyces avidinii. Addition streptavidin has improved sensitivity of the technique. It has a neutral isoelectric point that helps to decrease nonspecific binding to structures such as cell nuclei. Also, it does not contain carbohydrates present in avidin which might bind to tissue lecithin which is cause of nonspecific staining.

Labeled streptavidin-biotin (LSAB) method increased the sensitivity of immunostaining. It enables visualization of both polyclonal and monoclonal antibodies. This method has eliminated blocking step and reconfigured substrate chromogen reagents visualized using chromogen substrate.

Catalyzed Signal Amplification Method (CSA)

Tyramide signal amplification (TSA) is an enzyme mediated detection method which utilizes the catalytic activity of horseradish peroxidase (HRP) to generate high density labeling of a target protein or nucleic acid sequence in situ. This is based on principle of enzyme amplification was introduced by Bobrow et. al. for use of immunoblotting and ELISA assays. Later biotinylated tyramide was adapted to amplify immunohistochemical reactions on tissue sections (Adams et. al. 1992).

Horseradish peroxidase complex in presence of hydrogen peroxide catalyzes the biotynyl tyramide to form numerous free biotin sites. These reactive biotin radicals bind covalently to protein in the immediate vicinity of peroxidase enzymes. This reaction results in the deposition of numerous biotin signals will be captured by subsequent incubation with Streptavidin HRP complex that are then visualized with chromogenic substrate.

CSA II is biotin-free tyramide signal amplification system. This method is based on the peroxidase-catalyzed deposition of a fluoroscyl tyramide, followed by a secondary reaction with a peroxidase-conjugated anti-fluorescein which can be visualized by chromogen substrate. Use of fluoroscyl tyramide allows reducing background staining due to reactivity of endogenous biotin.

This method with introduction of polymer-based techniques is not used in routine diagnostic immunohistochemistry.

Polymer based Techniques—(Fig. 7.10)

The method is widely used technique in immunohistochemistry laboratory available on both manual and automated platforms. Polymer base techniques involve dextran polymer backbone to which multiple antibodies and enzyme molecules are conjugated. This eliminates nonspecific staining resulting from endogenous avidin biotin activity in tissues like liver, kidney and also can be used for tissues such as bone marrow, spleen, and frozen sections and also can impart well with double staining and multiplex staining. Polymer based two-step indirect technique uses an unconjugated

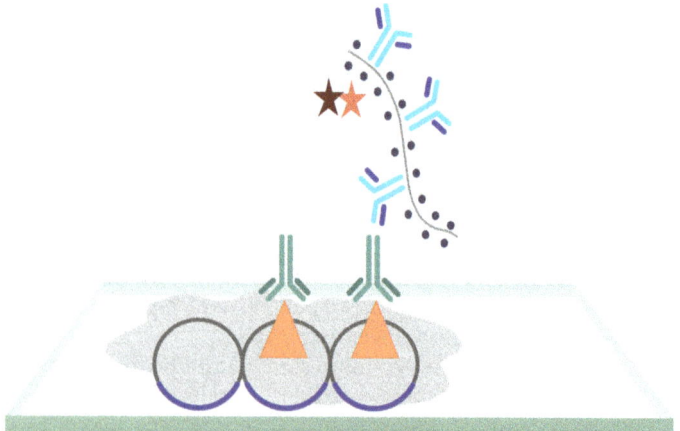

Fig. 7.10: Polymer based secondary antibody.

primary antibody followed by a secondary antibody conjugated to an enzyme (HRP) labeled dextran polymer chain. Conjugation of both anti-mouse and anti-rabbit secondary antibody allows same reagent to be used for monoclonal (rabbit and mouse) and polyclonal primary antibodies. This chain contains an average of 10 molecules of secondary antibody and 70 molecules of enzyme. Numerous companies have commercialized polymer-based systems which are method of choice for testing of immunostaining.

Newer detection kits have replaced dextran and other macromolecules with smaller polymers, micro polymers to increase access to the target antigen resulting in higher sensitivity, lower background and reduced nonspecific binding. When used polymer technique you may avoid using negative control.

In polymer technique two types of detection systems are available:
1. One step polymer detection system in which the polymer is tagged with secondary antibody and enzyme.
2. Two step polymer detection system in which the additional reagent is given as linker to enhance the signal (sensitivity) along with the secondary antibody tagged with HRP and polymer. Based on the research the two-step detection system is found to be more sensitive, specific, and recommended in majority of the nuclear markers.

Labels
Labels are molecules artificially attached to a protein which determines the amount of amplification and therefore the sensitivity of the technique.

- **Fluorescent labels**
  - Antibodies are tagged with fluorescent dyes and directly reacts with tissue antigen.
  - Commonly used fluorescent dyes are:
    - Fluorescein isothiocyanate (FITC)—Apple green color
    - Tetramethylrhodamine isothiocynate (TRITC)—Orange color
  - Immunofluorescence provides a rapid test, but final product is not permanent. The stains fade over a period of time.
- **Enzyme labels**: In this technique an unlabelled antibody serves as an antigen for a labeled secondary antibody with chromogen substrate gives stable, colored end product suitable for light microscopy and are suitable for frozen and paraffin section. The color of the end reaction varies depending on substrate and chromogen.
  - Horseradish peroxidase (HRP) is commonly used enzyme when used with:
    - 3, 3'Diaminobenzidine, DAB (Grahm and Karnovasky 1966) yields insoluble, dark brown end product.

- 3-amino-9-ethylcabazole, AEC: Rose red alcohol soluble end product.
- 4-chloro-1-naphthol (CN): Blue end product soluble in alcohol.
- Hanker-Yate's reagent: Blue black insoluble end product
- Calf alkaline phosphatase is used for the visualization of alkaline phosphatase activity. These methods are based on coupling of naphthol substrate, suitable azo dyes. Fast red TR, fast blue RR, and new fuchsin are chromogen dyes used. These dyes dissolve in alcohol hence slides cannot be mounted permanently.

  Use of multiple labels allow to identify two or more different antigens in the same tissue section. Alkaline phosphatase label is used sequentially with HRP.

- **Biotin:** A small vitamin molecule has great affinity to glycoprotein avidin that can be labeled with fluorochromes or enzymes.
- **Colloidal gold labels:**
  - Introduced by Faulk and Taylor.
  - Most popular metal tracer in use, exclusively in electron microscopy.
  - Method employs precipitation with silver ions which can be used to amplify the visibility of gold conjugates. Silver can also be used as conjugate and it gives a yellow color which is visible directly.

Chromogen

Results of an enzyme substrate reaction can be visualized by using chromogen. This produces colored end product which is suitable for light microscopy. Several different chromogens are available. **Diaminobenzidine (DAB)** is most commonly used chromogen substrate with horseradish peroxidase. DAB yields dark brown end products insoluble in alcohol, xylene and other organic solvents. DAB reaction can be intensified using imidazole, cupric sulfate etc. It can also be used for electron microscopy due to its electron dense nature. DAB is suspected carcinogen. Recently ready to use DAB is made commercially available, which has advantages of safety and less environmental pollution.

Refer to manufacturer's instruction for preparation protocol of DAB.

DAB is light sensitive chromogen. Once mixed with buffer, the working solution should store in dark.

Procedure for disposal of DAB:
- Excess reagent should be discarded properly.
- Mix DAB working solution with an equal volume of 20 % bleach.
- It is recommended that a copious amount of water be used to flush the drain after disposal of reagents.

Precautions:
- Avoid contact with skin
- Use of gloves is recommended.

Post-Chromogenic Enhancement

Another step that can noticeably improve the final result is post-chromogenic enhancement.

This involves placing the slides in a solution that enhances the positivity with DAB.

Copper sulfate 4% solution (25 mL vial), Sigma # C2284

To prepare, 5% solution—add one 25 mL vial to 175 mL of PBS (or 0.9% NaCl) in a staining dish.

The solution can be stored at room temperature for a month, and repeatedly re-used. To perform enhancement, place the staining dish in a 25°C oven, and incubate the slides for 1–5 minutes in the copper sulfate solution followed by running tap water and counterstaining with hematoxylin

Immunohistochemistry Staining—Total Test Approach

Success of immunohistochemistry test is dependent on performance of all steps in the staining protocol. Small errors in any of these steps may lead to false or inconsistent results.

Steps involved in total test approach:
- Tissue fixation
- **Test selection:** Understand need of IHC testing, selection of IHC markers, selection of paraffin block
- Selection and monitoring of appropriate control for test validation and daily QC
- Preparation and updation of control database and its application of daily QC

The preanalytical, analytical and post-analytical variables (**Table 7.1**) have a significant effect on the staining outcomes.

Preanalytical Phase

Any change in protocols may not directly relate to revalidation of the test, however any discrepancy comes across for the result from clinicians/oncologists, the preanalytical process needs to be validated and the need may arise for revalidation of IHC protocol for which, monitoring of preanalytical conditions is first step.

Tissue fixation

When tissue is removed from body it starts decomposing hence process of fixation should be prompt.

The time from excision of the specimen to the time the tissue is placed in the fixative (cold ischemic time) should be monitored.

Table 7.1: The preanalytical, analytical and post analytical variables.

Phases	Steps	Variables
Pre-analytical phase	Sample procurement	Delayed fixation, prolonged ischemia, thickness of sample
	Fixation	Cross-linking vs. coagulating fixatives, duration
	Decalcification	Type of decalcification solution and duration
	Tissue processing	Paraffin-embedded vs. frozen tissues
	Tissue sectioning	Thickness of tissue section, drying temperature and duration, tissue section aging
Analytical phase	Deparaffinization	Dewaxing agent
	Antigen retrieval	Detergents, enzymes, HIER
	Blocking non-specific reactivities	Endogenous enzymes, hydrophobic binding, pigments
	Primary antibodies	Monoclonal vs. polyclonal, Ag recognition (native vs. linear), specificity, species Variability
	Detection system	Avidin-biotin vs. polymer-based systems, ultrasensitive methods
	Enzyme-substrate-chromogen	Color detection
	Counter stain	Contrast between chromogen and counterstain
Post-analytical phase	Control performance	Animal species compatibility, tissue processing
	Interpretation	Pathologist vs. automated evaluation
	Report	Percentage of positive cells, positive vs. negative threshold, stand-alone test vs. ancillary test
		Diagnostic, prognostic test

This time should be as short as possible. Resected specimens like breast, lobectomy, gastrectomy, intestinal resection etc. should be sliced open for fixative to permeate it to avoid ischemic necrosis. The volume of fixative required is 15–20 times the volume of the tissue; container for the tissues must be appropriate to the size of the tissue.

College of American Pathologists (ASCO – CAP guidelines) has recommended that the tissue should be fixed minimum for 6 hours and maximum of 48 hours in 10% NBF [Neutral Buffered Formalin]

Fixative used, fixation time, cold ischemic time; in case bony specimens decalcifying fluid details and time of decalcification must be documented on requisition used at the time of gross examination.

Although fixation is paramount in the outcome of the antigen-antibody reaction, the incubation buffer and tissue-processing solutions can also alter antigenicity. The combination of cross-linking fixatives with heat and the nonpolar solvents used in paraffin embedding is thought to modify the antigen conformation **(Fig. 7.11)** so that specific epitopes may not be recognized by antibodies that would recognize those epitopes in frozen sections. Shifts in the tertiary structure of proteins (during processing) alter the structure of protein so that hydrophobic areas are oriented outward and hydrophilic regions inward (hydrophobic inversion) during dehydration and clearing steps, can reduce or abolish antibody binding without antigen retrieval especially with poorly stabilized (unfixed or sub optimally fixed in formalin) tissues/proteins exposed to a weakly polar or nonpolar solvent. This negative effect varies with the dehydrating and clearing agent used. There is also increased background reactivity in tissues left in xylene for prolonged periods during processing.

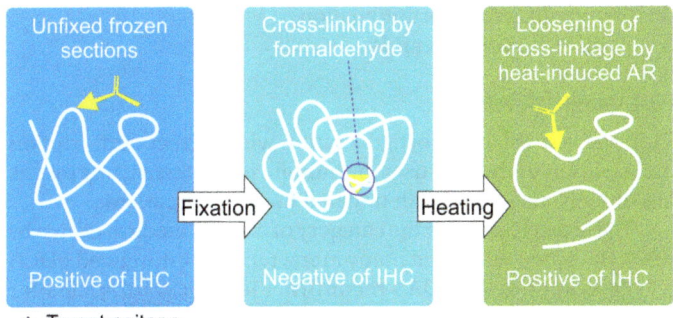

Fig. 7.11: Formaldehyde fixation can alter the 3-D structure of the epitope cross linkages; which is reversed by high temperature heating.

Analytical Phase

This phase involves immunohistochemistry staining process. (1) Antigen retrieval method (2) Selection of primary antibody (3) Detection system (4) Antibody validation.

The concept of IHC validation revolves around analytical phase. Revalidation in this phase will be applicable depending on results of daily controls. Validation of primary antibody is very important in immunohistochemistry for achieving accurate results.

Use of internal control is an ideal situation but, in each case, it is not possible to have internal controls.

In routine practice each test must accompany control and test tissue. This confirms the test performance.

Quality improvement criteria is applicable for:
- Validation of primary antibody
- Revalidation of lot-to-lot variation
- Buffers/diluents used

- Standardization with automation
- Positive/negative controls

Post Analytical Phase

This phase involves report generation with correct transcription and opinion of the end user. Immunohistochemistry test results are directly associated with targeted therapy for patients.

These tests belong to the category of class III medical device by FDA. He-2-neu, Alk-1 and many more; recently introduced PDL1.

Participation in EQAS reconfirms technical protocols for Immunohistochemistry.

Tissue Preparation

Post fixation tissues are processed (dehydration, clearing, infiltration, and finally embedded into paraffin wax) to produce paraffin block.

3–4 µm thin, uniform sections are cut; floated on warm water bath and then picked up slides. Remove any bubbles or wrinkles with a camel hair brush or teasing needle. Drain excess water by tilting slide on to blotting paper. Use positively charged slides for immunohistochemistry work up.

The important steps involved in any staining protocol:
- **Drying:** Slides are placed on hot plate or hot air oven to achieve adhesion.
- **Deparaffinization:** To remove paraffin from section, it is placed in xylene for 5 minutes and again for additional 5 minutes in another jar of xylene.
- **Hydration:** The slides are passed through decreasing concentrations of alcohol. Finally, these sections are washed in water, this ensures complete hydration of sections.

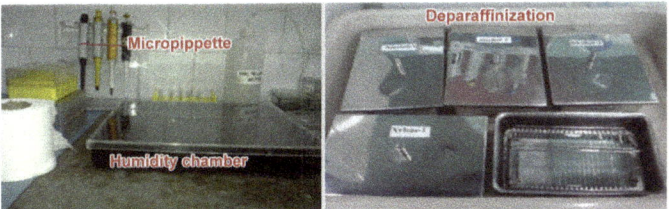

Fig. 7.12: Immunohistochemistry staining kit.

The process of paraffin section returning to water is referred as "Taking to water"

- **Staining:** It is carried out by the prescribed procedure **(Fig. 7.12)**
- **Post staining procedures**
  - After staining, the sections are rapidly agitated through grades of alcohol (dehydration) and two changes of xylene (clearing).
  - *Mounting:* This is carried out by placing a coverslip on the mounting medium laid over the specimen. Mounting slides protects tissue sections from dust and damage during storage and maintains refractive index necessary for microscopy.

Xylene and alcohol have to be replaced at regular interval. Patchy staining can be due to incomplete deparaffinization. Hazy sections can result because of less dehydration.

Automated staining equipment's have onboard facility for steps of pre and post staining protocols. Automatic cover slipper is considered as walk away system.

Positively Charged Slides

Tissue loss during immunohistochemical staining procedures may occur due to weak interaction of a tissue sample with glass surfaces.

The major reason of lifting of tissue is pretreatment protocol used for antigen retrieval. Many methods of adhering sections to the slides depend on using some material, usually protein, to act as contact glue between the glass and tissue. Most tissue sections in an aqueous medium, pH 5–7 carry negative charges. So, sections tend to adhere well to a glass slide if it is treated in such a way as to make it positively charged. Agents such as Poly-L-lysine, APES (Aminosilane) are routinely used in the laboratories. However, even with such surface modifications tissues subjected to HIER are lifted, folded, damaged or completely detached from slides after treatment have no control especially with IHC automation. Charged slides are different in that the adhesive compound has a positive charge and either coats the glass or bonds to it chemically. The positively charged coating attaches to the tissue through negative charges in the tissue and are hydrophilic in nature. These slides are commercially available (Matsunami Platinum pro)

Preparation of Poly-L-lysine Coated Slides

Poly-L-lysine is a commonly used basic polymer, having high pKa for an amino group and consequently Poly-L-lysine is positively charged even in moderately alkaline media. Poly-L-lysine is applied to slides as an aqueous solution, which is then allowed to dry by evaporations. This solution has been demonstrated as an effective tissue adhesive for use in various Heat mediated antigen retrieval protocol.

Reagent

- Poly–L-lysine, 0.1% w/v, in water (Sigma)
- 1% HCl
- Glass slides

Preparation

- Slides must be cleaned with 1% HCl before coating with Poly-L-Lysine
- Dilute Poly-L-lysine solution 1:10 with deionized water prior to coating slides
- Clean slides, a rack at a time in diluted solution for 5 minutes.
- Drain slides and dry in 60° oven for 1 hour or at room temperature overnight.
- Store in dust free boxes

Total 900 slides can be prepared with 100 mL (10×) of solution.

Note: There are numerous commercial positively charged slides available

Method for Overcoming Slide Hydrophobia

Milk treatment: Optional test to avoid impact of hydrophobic issue.

Dip slides in 20% of milk solution for 15–20 minutes before processing of slides for staining.

Antigen Retrieval (Figs. 7.13A and B)

Immunohistochemistry is routinely performed on FFPE. From before aldehyde is commonly used fixative worldwide. Fixation process preserves cells and tissue components in a "life like state" as possible.

Tissue antigens are masked during formalin fixation and paraffin wax processing. Formalin fixation causes cross links between antigens and unrelated proteins which are responsible in masking of tissue antigen which can prevent antigen antibody binding. This masking is known to form methylene bridges between reactive sites.

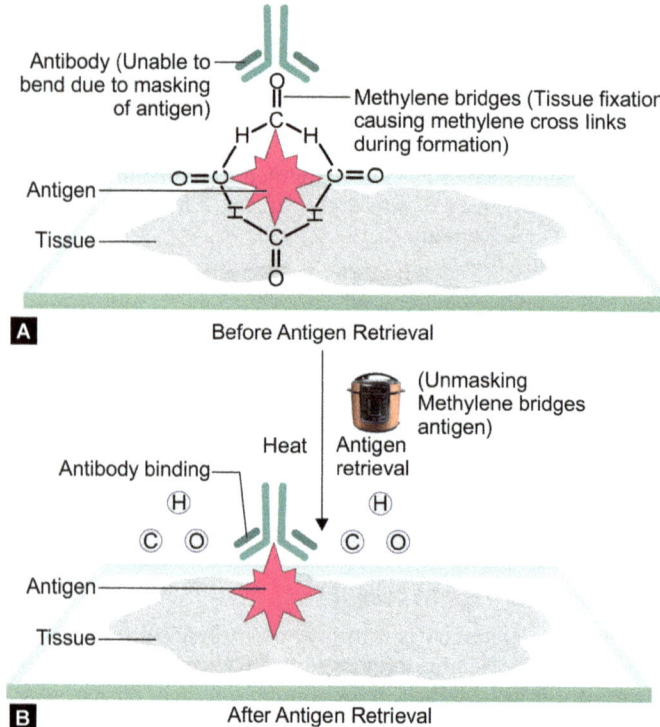

Figs. 7.13A and B: (A) Before antigen retrieval; (B) After antigen retrieval.

This cross link prevents primary antibody binding with antigenic sites. Various studies have suggested that the alteration caused by the formaldehyde fixation is reversible and that the antigens are unmasked. The technique involves use of proteolytic enzyme digestion or heat induced antigen retrieval methods. Antigen retrieval is pretreatment protocol for retrieving antigen from tissue sections back for immunostaining. Optimization of antigen retrieval is considered to be the important factor in achieving satisfactory results. Due to lack of standardization in tissue processing protocol, types of fixative used, duration of fixation, quality of sections cut there is no uniformity material used hence optimizing antigen retrieval protocol is challenging process.

Over-fixation, under-fixation
Over-fixation of tissues can produce false-negative results due to excessive cross-links, but the negative effects of over-fixation can often be reversed with an appropriate antigen retrieval procedure. The effects of over-fixation are somewhat dependent on the cellular location of the target antigen; over-fixation of nuclear antigens may not be reversible while cytoplasmic antigens may not be affected by over-fixation or can be recovered after antigen retrieval.

Under-fixation of tissues may result in cross-links forming only on the exterior of a sample and the center of the sample remaining unfixed. This can result in an inconsistent gradient of staining that is difficult to interpret. In addition, under-fixed tissues are more susceptible to damage or distortion caused by antigen retrieval methods.

Enzyme Digestion

The demonstration of many antigens was significantly improved by using various proteolytic enzymes like pepsin, trypsin, and protease. Duration of fixation has considerable effect on enzyme pretreatment. Therefore, the rules of standardization cannot be applied. However, with introduction of HMAR use of enzyme digestion protocol is limited to very few antibodies.

Length of enzyme digestion should be proportional to tissue exposure the fixative. However, time can be monitored using control tissue e.g., enzyme digestion for 1 minute, 2 minutes, 5 minutes... using titration methods.

Enzyme digestion can be used in combination with heat mediated retrieval methods.

Preparation

- **Pepsin:** 0.4% in 0.01 N HCl.
- **Pronase:** 0.05% in Tris buffer or Phosphate buffer pH 7.4
- **Trypsin:** 0.1% trypsin and 0.1 g of $CaCl_2$ in 100 mL of Tris or Phosphate buffer pH 7.4. Equilibrate solution at 37°C for ½ an hour.

Enzyme Pretreatment

- Place slides in humidity chamber for processing.
- Treat sections with desired enzyme
- The optimal time should be established by titration methods.

    For example,

Antibody dilution	Time in minutes
1:10	3, 5, 8 ...
1:20	3, 5, 8 ....
1:40	3, 5, 8 ....

    Antibody can be diluted serially and checked with different timings to achieve specific staining.
- Wash in running tap water to stop enzyme activity.
- Rinse in Wash buffer for 5 minutes.
- Continue with immunostaining.

Note
- ❖ Always prepare fresh enzyme solutions with each batch of staining.
- ❖ It is essential to monitor the digestion time at which the antigen is retrieved.
- ❖ For best results, the enzyme digestion time may be varied according to the enzyme utilized, its concentration, the fixation time, and tissue type, thickness of the sections, and specific antigen to be tested.

Heat Mediated Antigen Retrieval (HMAR)

The use of heat to unmask antigens has increased the number of antibodies that can be used on paraffin sections. Unmasking antigen is possible by exposing tissue sections to high temperature; it definitely helps to break or alter protein cross linkage caused by formaldehyde. Heating time and temperature, pH of retrieval solution used have effect on the final results. There is no single retrieval solution that is best for all antigens. Different methods can be used for HMAR technique.

Factors influencing HMAR (Fig. 7.14)

- ❖ **Heating time and temperature:** Heating time and heating temperature have inverse proportion:
  - Higher temperature less heating time
  - Lower temperature longer heating time
  - Studies have shown on heating tissue section produces hydrolysis which leads to break down of cross linkages formed during fixation.
- ❖ **pH of buffer solutions:** Higher pH of buffer solution (Tris-EDTA buffer pH 9.0) is suitable for the majority of the antibodies.

Chapter 7: Immunohistochemistry

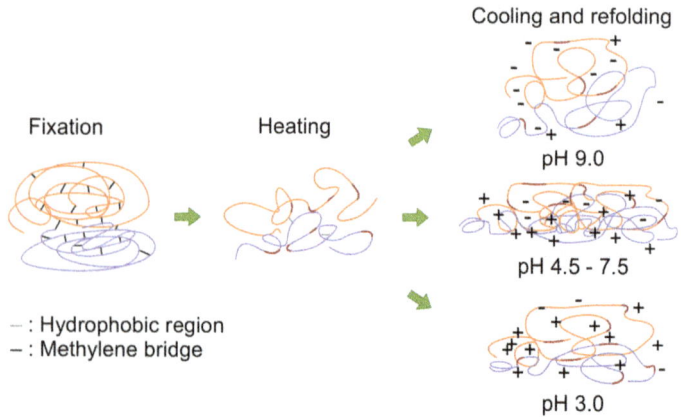

Effect of heat induced epitope retrieval at different pH of the retrieval buffer.
  After heating, methylene bridges produced by formaldehyde are cleaved and polypeptide chains extended to expose their hydrophobic regions. During cooling process, the polypeptide chains rapidly refold. At pH 3.0 and pH. 0.0, hydrophobic attractive force and electrostatic repulsion force based on positively or negatively charged polypeptides may balance to prevent intertwining of polypeptide chains and expose antigenic determinants for antigen-antibody interaction. On the other hand, at pH 4.5–7.5, ionic and hydrophobic attractive forces may cooperatively act, and neighboring polypeptides entangle each other to hidden antigenic determinants.

Fig. 7.14: Heating time and temperature.

Microwave Oven (Fig. 7.15)

Various studies have shown improved immunohistochemical staining by use of microwave irradiation. This technique was

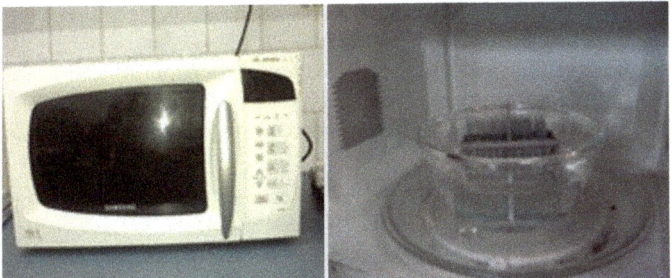

Fig. 7.15: Microwave oven.

developed by Dr Shan-Rg Shi and colleagues. Initially the tissue sections were dipped in solutions of heavy metals like lead thiocyanate, zinc sulfate. Later, the heavy metals were replaced by 0.01 M citrate buffer (pH 6.0). The majority of antigens gave excellent results with microwave heating for 10–30 minutes. Due to uneven heat, the results can be inconsistent when large batches of slides are used. Large volume of buffer and rotating trays can be used to reduce this effect. Domestic microwave ovens and laboratory microwave models are used.

Domestic Microwave Oven Pretreatment

- After deparaffinization slides are placed in microwave resistant plastic jar containing desired antigen retrieval buffer.
- Cover the jars with loose fitting covers and heat in microwave oven.
- For 10 to 30 minutes, at desired temperature depending on antibody used (5 minutes × number of cycles).

- With an interval of 1 minute in between the cycles to check the fluid levels.
- Add distilled water to the jars to compensate for the quantity of buffer lost during microwaving after each cycle.
- After heating cool the slides in coupling jar containing citrate buffer for 20 minutes.
- Wash the slides in Wash buffer for 5 minutes.
- Continue immunostaining in the usual way.

Pressure Cooker/Autoclave

Pressure cooker/autoclave has been considered as an alternative to microwave oven. Sections are boiled in desired antigen retrieval buffer under pressure. Various studies have proved that pressure cooker is also efficient like microwave. Antigen unmasking is consistent even with the larger batches of slides. They are simple to use, and have the advantage to produce heat up to 120°C without significant loss of buffer.

Temperature/time controlled programmable pressure cooker models are available.

Pressure Cooker Pretreatment (Fig. 7.16)

- Use a 5-liter capacity stainless steel domestic pressure cooker.
- Boil 3 liters of 0.01 M citrate buffer PH 6.0 in the pressure cooker, but not under the pressure. When the buffer is boiling, place the slides is place in the buffer. Close the pressure cooker lid and bring to full pressure. Then boil for 2 minutes. Timing starts only when full pressure is reached.
- After boiling, cool the pressure cooker under running tap water until pressure is released.

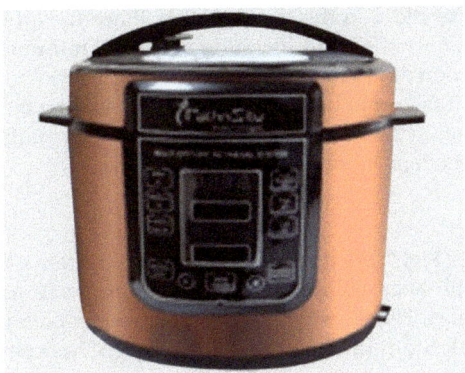

Fig. 7.16: Pressure cooker.

- Remove the slides from cooker and quickly wash in running tap water and transfer to wash buffer. Do not allow slides to dry.

Pretreatment for Programmable Pressure Cooker
- This cooker has programmable temperature; 125°C for 30 seconds and 90°C for 10 seconds.
- Remove the slides from cooker and cool at room temperature for 20 minutes.
- **Water bath:** Conventional water bath can be used for antigen retrieval. Temperature just below the boiling point of water 95-99°C is adequate.

Pretreatment
- Preheat water bath with staining dish containing retrieval buffer until temperature reaches 95–100°C.

- ❖ Immerse slides in the staining dish. Place the lid loosely on the staining dish and incubate for 20–40 minutes (optimal incubation time should be determined by user).
- ❖ Turn off the water bath and remove the staining dish to room temperature and allow the slides to cool for 20 minutes.
- ❖ Rinse sections in wash buffer for 5 minutes.

PT Module

PT module (**Fig. 7.17**) is automated retrieval system which avails facility of preheat temperature, retrieval temperature and cool down settings. These systems are based on water bath principles.

PT Link module heats the slides at 97°C temperature for 20 minutes.

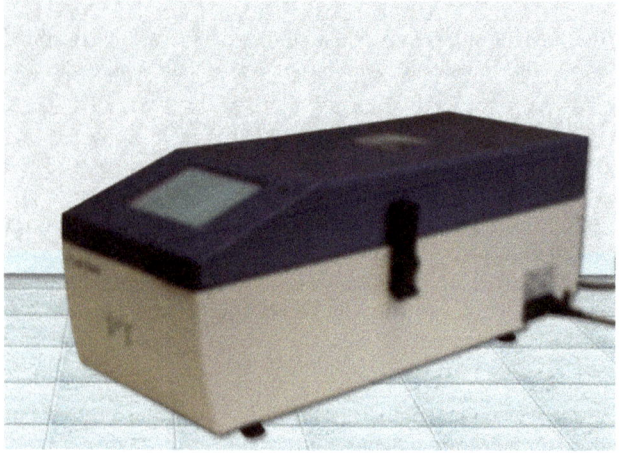

Fig. 7.17: PT module.

Note
- ❖ It is advisable for each laboratory to evaluate different epitope retrieval systems/solutions and choose those that work best for the particular antigens of interest.
- ❖ Always keep the same number of incubation jars filled with fluid in the microwave oven/pressure cooker at all the times, even if small batches of slides are to be processed. This will maintain consistency in the heating runs.

Commonly used buffers are
- ❖ Tris buffer saline is used as WASH buffer
- ❖ Sodium citrate buffer pH 6.0
- ❖ Tris EDTA buffer pH 9.0

Preparation of Buffers

Today antigen retrieval and wash buffers are available commercially along with detection kits. However, composition of buffers is given for reference.

- ❖ *Tris buffer 0.05 M pH 7.6 (stock)*
  Dissolve 6.1 g Tris in 50 mL of distilled water.
  Add 38 mL of 1N HCl.
  Dilute to total volume of one liter with distilled water at pH 7.6 +/- 0.2.
  Store the solution at room temperature.
  For large workload concentrated (10×) can be prepared and diluted 1:10 before use. Always check the pH of buffer before use
- ❖ *Tris buffer saline (TBS)*

0.05 M Tris buffer	100 mL
0.85% NaCl	900 mL

This buffer can be used as wash buffer in staining procedure. 0.05% Tween 20 can be added to wash buffer to reduce background staining.

- *Phosphate buffer saline (PBS) 0.01 M, pH 7.2*

Dibasic sodium phosphate anhydrous ($Na_2 HPO_4$)	1.48 g
Monobasic potassium phosphate anhydrous ($KH_2 PO_4$)	0.43 g
Sodium Chloride	7.2 g

  Dilute to total volume of one liter with distilled water.
  PBS can be used as Wash buffer

- *Citrate buffer 0.01M pH 6.0*

  Stock solution A—0.1 M Citric acid
  2.1 grams of citric acid dissolved one litre of distilled water
  Stock solution B—0.1 M sodium citrate
  2.91 grams of sodium citrate dissolved in one liter of distilled water.
  Working solution: 9 mL of A + 41 mL of B. Add distilled water to final volume 500 mL.
  Prepare working solution FRESH.

- *Tris-EDTA buffer (0.01 M Tris, 1mM EDTA, pH 9.0)*

Tris	1.21 g
EDTA	0.37 g
Distilled water	1,000 mL

  (Stock can be prepared as 10×. Final volume must be 100 mL to make 10×)

Antibody Validation

Validation of primary antibody is very important in immunohistochemistry for achieving accurate results. The concept of validation revolves around analytical phase.

Validation is the action of checking or proving the validity or accuracy of the any process.

In immunohistochemistry whether an antibody recognizes the correct protein based on cellular localization is validated.

Purpose of validation of antibody in immunohistochemistry is to measure
- Sensitivity
- Specificity
- Reproducibility
- Accuracy

Guidelines for validation of new antibody are defined wherein; 10–20 different tissues for positive and negative controls are to be tested.

Validation of new IHC markers, revalidation of existing antibodies, quality monitoring on a daily basis are a few compulsory tasks in immunohistochemistry processes. The results are based on a comparison of controls and tests.

It is essential to determine optimal titers of all primary antibodies before putting them into diagnostic use. All antibodies are to be tested on known positive and negative antigen containing tissues.

Primary Antibody

Antibodies are available commercially with different pack size as ready to use (RTU) or concentrated.

Ready to use (RTU) antibodies are diluted optimally by manufacturer and can be used directly as per recommendation using appropriate controls. RTU antibodies are easy to use for beginners.

Concentrated antibodies are supplied with recommended dilutions by manufacturer and is economical solution for IHC labs with large workload.

Antibody Description

Manufacturer's recommendations sheet **(Table 7.2)** is received along with pack of primary antibody contains specification of antibodies such as, *Ref. Datasheet of Vimentin*

Table 7.2: Manufacturer's recommendations sheet.

Staining recommendations

Antigen retrieval solution	• Use EDTA Buffer (PathnSitu Cat # PS008) as antigen retrieval solution • **Heat retrieval method:** Retrieve sections under steam pressure for 15 min using PathnSitu's multi epitope retrieval system then allow solution to cool for 10 minutes then transfer tissue sections/slides to distilled water
Primary antibody	• Cover the tissue sections with primary antibody and incubate for 30 minutes at room temperature when used PathnSitu PolyExcel detection system
Detection system	• Refer to PathnSitu PolyExcel detection system protocol or manufacturer's detection kit staining protocol when used other vendor detection system.
Cellular localization	• Cytoplasm
Positive control	• Uterine leiomyoma, colon, appendix
Troubleshooting	• Follow the antibody specific protocol recommendations according to the data sheet provided. If unusual results occur, contact PathnSitu technical support at 040- 2701 5544 or techsupport@pathnsitu.com

Limitations and warranty: There are no warranties, expressed or implied, which extend beyond this description. PathnSitu is not liable for property damage, personal injury, or economic loss caused by this product.

Bibliography:
1. Skalli O, et al. J Cell Biol.1986 Dec; 103(6 Pt 2): 2787-96.
2. Roholl PJ, et al. Hum Pathol.1990 Dec;21(12):1269-74.
3. Raymond W, et al. Pathology.1991 Oct;23(4):291-7.

- **Source:** Mouse monoclonal/rabbit monoclonal/polyclonal
- Monoclonal antibodies are labeled with Clone e.g., E29, SP3,
- **Isotope:** IgG or IgM
- List of known positive and known negative normal and tumor tissues
- Protein concentration, suggested working dilution ranges.
- **Pretreatment protocol:** Antigen retrieval method, pH of buffer used, time, temperature.
- **Storage conditions:** Helps to maintain antibody stability and maximum reactivity for the life of antibody i.e., expiration date
- Intended use such as antibody is in vitro use (IVD), research use only (RUO) or analyte specific reagent (ASR)
- These are to be considered only as guidelines for the validation protocol.
- Also, guidelines for antibody description, assessment, and recommended protocol and tissue preparation is available on http://www.nordiqc.org

Selection of Controls

Select appropriate control block for the antibody to be validated.

Guidelines for control tissues, tissue preparation are available on, http://www.pathologyoutlines.com
www.Ihcworld.com
http://www.nordiqc.org
Ref. Http://www.Pathologyoutlines.Com *Primary antibody CA 125*

Criteria for Selection of Blocks for Validation (Table 7.3)

Positive Control

- The tissue section that contains representing target antigen which gives definite positive reaction also, must possess low levels of antigen expression as is often seen in tumor tissue. Exclusive use of normal tissues that have high-levels of antigen expression may result in antibody titers of insufficient sensitivity will lead to false negative results. For validation of antibody known positive tissue block has to be selected from both normal and tumor tissue containing desired antigen.
- If positive control does not perform, the test must be considered as invalid. This confirms false negative staining.
- Ideally, the positive control should always be processed in the same manner as the test section.
- Positive control defines technical sensitivity and specificity of immunostaining protocol.
- A positive control section included on the same slide as the patient tissue is optimal practice.

Table 7.3: Criteria for selection of blocks for validation.

Positive staining-normal

Fetus: Amnion, coelomic and mullerian epithelium (Asia Oceania J Obstet Gynaecol 1990:16:379)

Adults: Mesothelial cells and luminal surface of epithelial cells of endocervix, endometrium, fallopian tube; also, in small amounts in epithelium of apocrine sweat glands, biliary tract, colon, mammary gland, pancreas, stomach

Positive staining-disease

Carcinomas of biliary tree, breast, cervix, endometrium, fallopian tubes, liver, lung, ovary (serous, usually not mucinous), pancreas: ovarian sex cord tumors

Aveolar rhabdomyosa'cama of uterus, desmoplastic small round cell tumor of pelvic peritoneu m, epithelioid sarcoma (Arch Pathnol Lab Med 2006:130:871. Jpn J Clin Oncol 2004:34:149). Intralobar pulmonary sequestration (Intern Med 2002:41:875). Leiomyoma of ileal mesentery, mesothelioma, seminal vessel adenocarcinoma

Endometrosis (Hum Pathol 2008:39:954), Inflammatory disorderes, leiomyomas of ileal mesentery, pregnancy

Negative staining

* Normal ovary, squamous cells

Negative Control

A tissue section which lacks the tissue representing target antigen. This control helps in detecting/eliminating unintended antibody cross reactivity to the cells or cellular components or unintended background staining.

- ❖ A known negative tissue block is selected from tissue which does not represent the desired antigen OR This can be achieved by omitting the primary antibody and replacing it with buffer or nonimmune serum from the same species of primary antibody.

- One negative control must be processed for each block of patient tissue being immunostained.
- Polymer-based detection systems (biotin-free) are sufficiently free from background reactivity to obviate the need for a negative reagent control in immunostaining and such controls may be omitted at discretion of the laboratory director following appropriate validation (CAP checklist). However, with the tissue containing pigments use of negative control will be of help.

Internal control **is referred as "built in control" or "in-house control" (Figs. 7.18A and B).**

The target antigen is visualized within normal tissue elements. Ideally positive control must be processed similar to the test, but it is always not possible. One can select positive control in the same tissue section which is in adjacent normal elements. *For example, smooth muscle actin in stomach; p40 in cervix stains squamous epithelium and negative in tumor cells.*

Vimentin is also referred as internal control, which is present in almost all tissue sections and sensitive for fixation and processing. Vimentin can identify optimally fixed and processed tissue. If it shows weak staining tissue is thought to be over fixed. Hence Battifora refers to Vimentin as "Reporter molecule."

Cell Line Controls (Figs. 7.19A and B)

Cell line controls are independent external reference controls used for validation and evaluation. These are available with FDA approved kits for companion diagnostics like Her-2-neu, Alk-1, EGFR, c-kit.

Different FDA approved 'kits' include sections of FFPE cell line pellets, e.g., HercepTest (negative, low and high positive)

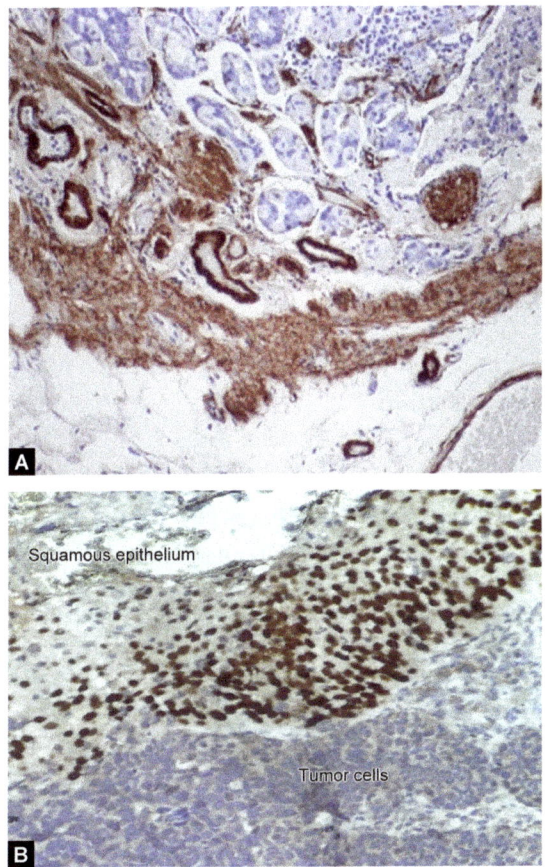

Figs. 7.18A and B: Internal control: (A) Internal control—smooth muscle actin in stomach; (B) Internal control -p40 in cervix.

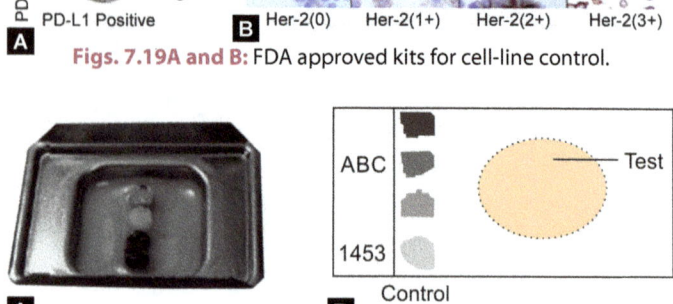

Figs. 7.19A and B: FDA approved kits for cell-line control.

Figs. 7.20A and B: Multitumor tissue block.

Multitumor Tissue Blocks (Figs. 7.20A and B)

The technique evolved by Dr Hector Battifora.

"Use of multitumor paraffin blocks is a key to effective and efficient validation IHC laboratory" *refer* to CAP guidelines.

This will be of great help for validation of primary antibodies of predictive and nonpredictive assays.

10 positive and 10 negative control sections for validation of nonpredictive assay.

Tissues processed and infiltrated in paraffin are used for preparation of multitumor blocks. Selected tissue blocks can be melted by keeping on hotplate. Tissues can be cut into small bit small bits using blade. These bits are remolded again in new mold. Place small bits of tissue vertically side by side in the bottom of embedding mold.

One has to be careful while mounting as different types of tissues are selected, they have to be arranged in a row, at identical level. Biopsy punch needle with plunger **(Fig. 7.21)** will be of great help for preparation multitumor paraffin blocks. Tissue microarray kits **(Fig. 7.22)** are also commercially available.

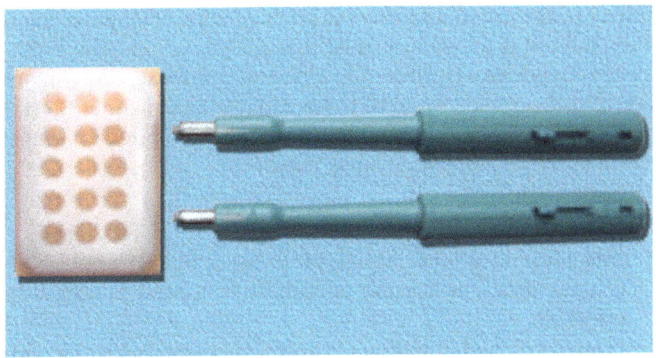

Fig. 7.21: Biopsy punch needle with plunger.

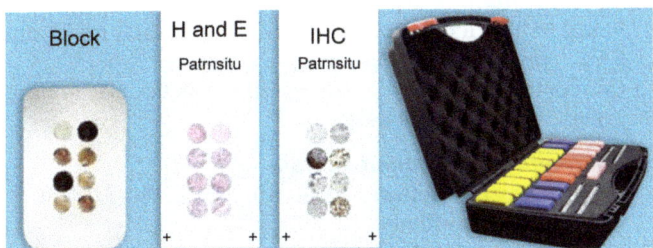

Fig. 7.22: Tissue microarray kits.

Different mixtures of tissues such as appendix, skin, tonsil, skeletal muscle, liver, and pancreas can be selected for the same. Known positive tumor tissues such as melanoma, Hodgkin's lymphoma, ALK 1 positive lymphoma, hormones can be selected for control database.

Multitumor block can be used as a positive control for any stain that is desired. Sections can be precut and placed at one end. Slides can be stored and used as positive control when in need. When the test is to be performed tissue is placed on other end of already cut positive control slide. Test and control sections on one slide allow both sections to be stained in identical manner. Storing recut slides at room temperature is not recommended for longer period as tissue antigenicity may be affected.

Responsibility

- Selection and monitoring of appropriate control is responsibility of pathologist who is reporting authority of the test for diagnostic purposes.
- Preparation and updation of control database and application of daily controls is responsibility of technologist.

Method for validation of primary antibody
- Ready to use (RTU) antibodies are available as 1 mL, 3 mL, 6 mL, 7 mL, and 12 mL pack size.
- Concentrated antibodies are available as 0.1 mL, 0.2 mL, 0.5 mL, 1 mL, 2 mL pack size.

Basic formula to understand dilution
- **Range of micropipettes:** 1–10 µL, 10–100 µL, 100–1,000 µL
- **Concentrated antibody:**

0.1 mL = 100 µL
1.0 mL = 1,000 µL

Check with dilution suggested in datasheet given by manufacturer. Dilute antibody using serial dilution, for e.g., 1:10 i.e., 1 µL antibody + 9 µL antibody diluent using appropriate micropipette. Serial dilution is the process of taking a sample and diluting it with desired diluent.

For e.g., if recommended dilution is 100 to 500.

Define number of dilutions to be performed for validation of primary antibody.

1:100, 1:200, 1:400, 1:500, 1: 600

RTU antibody: 6 mL = 6000 µL; if 100 µL of antibody is used per slide 6,000/100 = 60 tests can be performed in 6 mL RTU.

- 1st run of serial dilution is checked with no antigen retrieval.
- 2nd run of serial dilution is checked with antigen retrieval protocol.
- Different antigen retrieval protocols such as enzyme digestion, heat mediated antigen retrieval (HMAR) using pressure cooker, microwave, water bath, PT link.
- Different antigen retrieval buffers—citrate buffer, Tris EDTA buffer etc.
- Define best antigen retrieval protocol for antibody validation.
- Evaluate staining results to decide which optimal titer of antibody and precise antigen retrieval protocol is effective.
- If e.g., 1:100 dilution gives weak staining with no nonspecific staining then go with the more concentrated dilution such as 1:25, 1:50, … but if 1:100 dilution gives strong staining with background stain then dilute further 1:200, 1: 300……
- Document antibody validation protocol and results **(Table 7.4)**.

Table 7.4: Validation of new antibody.

VALIDATION OF NEW ANTIBODY

NAME OF ANTIBODY -   DATE -
CLONE –
VENDOR –
PACK SIZE -   REF -   LOT NO -   EXPIRY DATE
DILUTION RECOMMENDED BY MANUFACTURER -
DETECTION SYSTEM-

VALIDATION CHART

METHOD FOR ENZYME RETRIEVAL -HIER - PH

Sr. no.	Block no.	Tissue	Dilution	Remarks

TEST DONE BY   PATHOLOGIST

- ❖ Documentation must include antibody lot, expiry date, primary antibody, dilutions, blocking, link antibody, label, chromogen used, incubation time, incubation temperature, retrieval method.
- ❖ Antigen antibody reaction can be viewed with the different staining pattern such as nuclear, cytoplasmic, and membranous.

- Validation report must be duly signed by pathologist.
- Each new batch of antibody, detection system and chromogen must be checked for reactivity and documented. The new lot of staining must be compared with existing lot in use.
- Controls are to be reviewed at least monthly to detect trends.

CAP GUIDELINES—ANP.22750 Antibody Validation REVISED** 07/28/2015

Means of validation may include, but are not limited to:
- Correlating the results using the new antibody with the morphology and expected results; comparing the results using the new antibody with the results of prior testing of the same tissues with a validated assay in the same laboratory.
- Comparing the results using the new antibody with the results of testing the same tissue in another laboratory with a validated assay; or
- Comparing the results using the new antibody with previously validated non-IHC tests or testing previously graded tissue challenges from a formal proficiency testing program.
- For an initial validation, laboratories should achieve at least 90% overall concordance between the new test and the comparator test or expected results.

For validation of a nonpredictive assay, the validation should test a minimum of 10 positive and 10 negative tissues.

For validation of predictive markers (with the exception of HER2, ER and PgR), the laboratory should test a minimum of 20 positive and 20 negative tissues.

In either situation, when the laboratory director determines that fewer validation cases are sufficient for a specific marker (e.g., a rare antigen or tissue), the rationale for that decision needs to be recorded. Positive cases in the validation set should span the expected range of clinical results (expression level), especially for those markers that are reported quantitatively.

The laboratory director is responsible for determining the number of positive and negative cases and the number of predictive and nonpredictive markers to test.

Also refer to Summary of Guideline from the College of American Pathologists Pathology and Laboratory Quality Center – Total 14 recommendations visit site https://www.cap.org/

Standard Staining Protocol (Fig. 7.23)

Method

- 3 µm thick sections are mounted on slides coated with adhesives and fixed in incubator for overnight at 37°C or incubate at 60°C for 1 hour.
- Deparaffinize sections in xylene and graded of alcohol to water.
- Quench endogenous peroxidase activity. Incubate slide in hydrogen peroxide block for 10 minutes.
- Rinse in buffer wash for 5 minutes.
- Perform antigen retrieval step as desired either using enzymes or heat mediated protocols.
- Rinse in buffer wash for 5 minutes.
- Incubate with "blocking serum" for 5 minutes; check manufacturer's recommendations.
- Rinse in buffer wash. This step can be optional
- Incubate with primary antibody for 1 hour at room temperature; check manufacturer's recommendations.
- Rinse in buffer wash for 10 minutes; 2 changes of 5 minutes each.
- Incubate with secondary link antibody (HRP polymer) for 20 to 30 minutes; check manufacturer's recommendations.

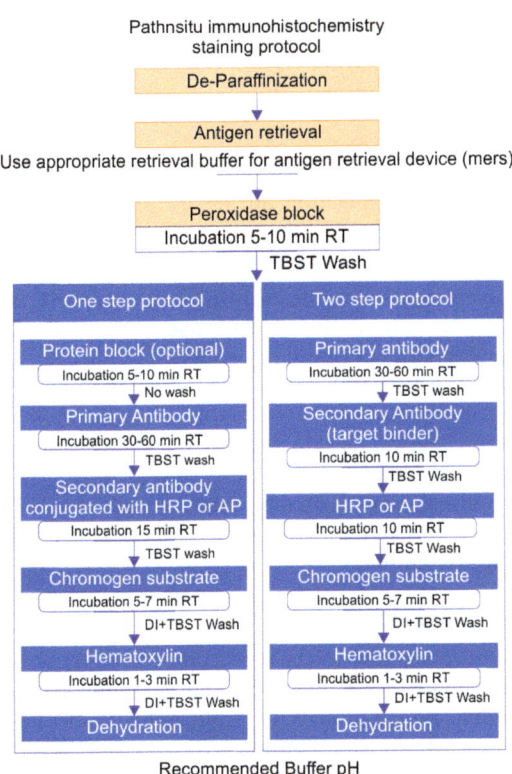

Fig. 7.23: Staining protocol.

- Rinse in buffer wash for 10 minutes; 2 changes of 5 minutes each
- Apply chromogen substrate for 5 to 10 minutes; incubation time needs to be optimized.
- Rinse in distilled water for 5 minutes
- Counter stain with hematoxylin
- Rinse in running tap water
- Dehydrate, clear and cover slip using DPX.

Immunohistochemistry on Cytology (ICC) Smears

Studies have proved correlation of ICC with tissue IHC results.

- Previously stained smears can also be used for staining; destaining of smears is not necessary.
- Smears can be dried thoroughly after fixation to achieve excellent results.
- Common fixatives used in cytology are ether/alcohol, ethanol, methanol and acetone.
- Adherence of the cells on the smear is excellent
- Immunostaining on cytology smears show minimum nonspecific staining

Specimen Preparation

Immunohistochemistry can be performed on cell blocks, FNAC—fragments of tissue, direct smears, cytocentrifuge preparation, Liquid based cytology preparation. When sufficient fluid specimens of all types particularly effusions, endometrial aspirates, brush smears as well as fine needle aspirates are available cell blocks can be prepared. Concept of positive, negative control; control database is applicable to cell block preparation for immunohistochemistry staining.

Preparation of Cell Block

Ethanol formalin is a fixative used for processing cell block. This fixative results in excellent cytomorphological features that closely resemble the cytologic detail seen in Papanicolaou stained smears. Preservation of histochemical and immunocytochemical properties are preserved.

The fixative must be prepared fresh and used immediately because formalin is capable of oxidizing to formic acid.

Preparation

37 to 40% formaldehyde	100 mL
95% ethanol	900 mL

Method

- Fix the smears in cytological fixative for half an hour.
- Stain the smears with routine PAP or H&E stain.
- Scan the slides and mark the area suitable for staining.
- Remove cover slip by passing through xylene and alcohol.
- Do not destain the slides.
- Proceed with immunohistochemistry staining protocol.

Quality Control for Immunostaining for Cytology

In cytology need to establish a bank of imprints or frozen cells from normal and neoplastic cells containing antigen of interest. Also, database for negative for the antigen. Negative control can be performed by omitting the primary antibody and replacing it with buffer or nonimmune serum of the same species of primary antibody.

If a single slide is available, portions of the same slide can be used as test and negative controls by marking areas with a diamond pencil. Method of specificity is best determined by using negative control. Control cell lines are also used for quality control in immunostaining of cytology smears.

Multiple Staining in Immunohistochemistry

"Simultaneous visualization of multiple markers on single tissue section". This method allows visualization of two or more proteins at different location in one tissue section.

For example, Kapa/Lambda chains, PIN 4 consists of a cocktail of three antibodies including AMACR, p63 and high molecular weight cytokeratin; Desmoglein 3+ p40+ Napsin and many more.

Method selection criteria:
- Primary antibodies made in different species rabbit/mouse
- It is important to eliminate any cross reactivity between reagents

Staining Method

Sequential staining: One staining method is followed by another; for example:
Step 1—Tissue + primary antibody (first)
Step 2—Peroxidase conjugated polymer (first)
Step 3—Chromogen substrate (first)
Step 4—Double stain block
Step 5—Primary antibody (second)
Step 6—Alkaline phosphatase conjugated polymer (second)
Step 7—Chromogen substrate (second)

This method allows avoiding problems related to cross reactivity, but it cannot be used for colocalized targets. This technique has often has long-standing protocol.

Simultaneous staining: The primary antibody can be applied simultaneously. Directly labeled antibody or an unlabeled primary antibody raised in different host species can be used. This is less time consuming than sequential method but needs to keep check on cross reactivity.

Micro polymer detection kits are now commercially available for multiple staining protocol. Alkaline phosphatase (AP) and horseradish peroxidase (HRP) micro polymer technology is designed for detecting multiple antigens on same tissue section.

Automation in Immunohistochemistry

Automation in immunohistochemistry as eased the technician's job, improve quality. Inter laboratory comparison and reproducibility of results is achievable.

Two types of autostainers are available.
1. **Semi-automatic:** These equipments have facility to stain slides after antigen retrieval. Deparaffinization and antigen retrieval steps are performed outside the equipment stages 1, 2, 4). ONLY stage 3 is performed in the system. Equipment will take care of only staining but can be definitely of great to reduce efforts in manual staining.
2. **Fully automatic:** Slides are placed in the stainer immediately after sectioning. Automatic stainers have facility to execute complete processing of slides from drying to counter stain and continuous batch processing.

Automation has also provided centralized slide programming by connecting equipment to the computer. The number of equipment's attached to the computer varies from 3 to 8 depending on the software used.

Working Principle

Capillary Gap Technique

Technique employed in auto stainer is capillary gap principle, distance between multiple slides, volume of primary/secondary antibody, gaps of washing.

Numbers of slides are defined in the system. The capillary gap retains defined amount of fluid by surface tension and excess is automatically overflows and drained out. This prevents drying of sections during subsequent steps. Use of cover tiles in the system prevents air bubble formation on slide. Cover tile is placed on one end of slide.

Liquid Cover Slip Method

Special oil is used in the auto stainer to cover the slides which prevents drying of reagents throughout the staining process. This technique is known as liquid cover slip method. These systems are specifically designed to work at high temperature.

Leica Bond max; Caliber 30 has cover tile methodology and central host computer for 5 equipment's and Roche Bench XT utilizes liquid cover slip method and central host computer for 8 equipments.

Both are fully automated systems.

Trouble Shooting

The ideal end result of immunostaining is expected to be specific, accurate, and reproducible.

Hallmarks of Ideal Immunostaining (Fig. 7.24)

Strong, crisp staining on target cells with no diffusion in surrounded tissue, no staining + cross reactivity in nontarget cells, correct contrast with counter stain

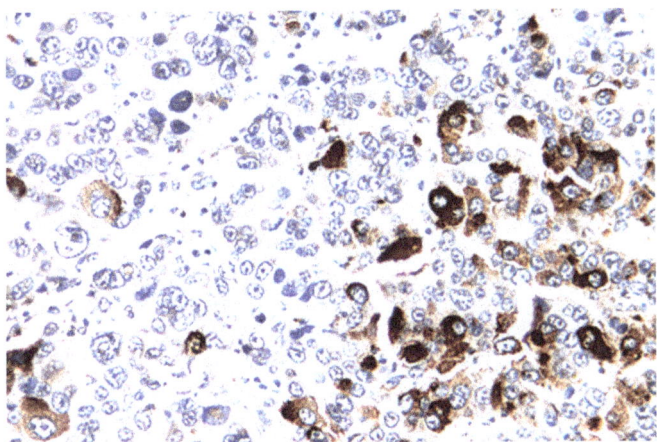

Fig. 7.24: Strong, crisp staining—alpha-fetoprotein—hepatocellular carcinoma.

Many factors such as fixation, tissue processing, antigen retrieval, buffers, detection systems, antibodies, storage conditions are responsible for specific staining with no background. Sometimes due to over staining with counter stain, tissues getting detached from slide will result in shabby appearance of immunohistochemistry preparation. Any variation in protocol can result in no staining or weak staining, over staining, background in the tissue section. Adhere to guidelines referred to in manufacturer's data sheet; staining pattern of each primary antibody is defined **(Figs. 7.25A to C)**.

Chapter 7: Immunohistochemistry

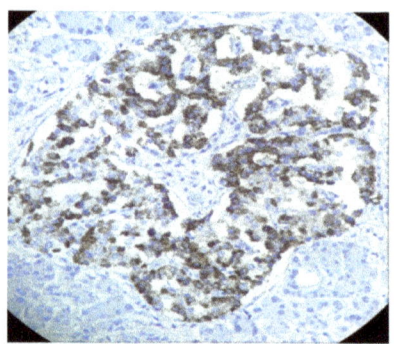

A Chromagranin A-islets of pancreas

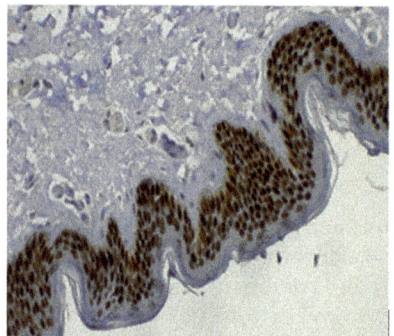

B p40 positive; squamous cells; skin

Figs. 7.25A and B

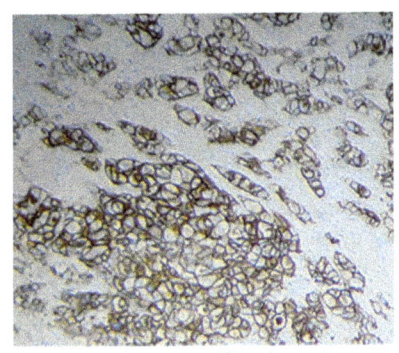

C Her-2-new positive; breast

Figs. 7.25A to C: Defined staining pattern of primary antibody.

For example, chromogranin A—cytoplasm, p40- nuclei, Her-2-Neu—membrane.

Background

Background staining can be caused by incorrect antibody binding.

Endogenous Enzyme Activity

Endogenous Peroxidase

Endogenous enzymes are present in a variety of cells and tissue types. Red blood cells, placenta, Endogenous peroxidase blocks prevent an enzyme that originates within a cell or tissue from causing a reaction with another substance or substrate. Peroxidase activity is the result of the decomposition of hydrogen peroxidase. This results in false positive staining.

Incubation with 0.3% H_2O_2/methanol for 10–30 minutes is enough to achieve required results. In the case of frozen sections, methanol cannot be used due to its fixation properties and 0.3% H_2O_2 must be used instead.

Endogenous Alkaline Phosphatase

Endogenous alkaline phosphatase activity is present in intestine, kidney, liver, bone cells, blood in varied amount.

Including 5 mM levamisole in chromogen substrate solution will help to quench endogenous alkaline phosphatase.

In paraffin sections usually the activity is lost during processing. In double staining enzyme substrates need to quench both endogenous peroxidase and alkaline phosphatase activities. The sequence of blocking is optional. Reagents that block both in a single step are available.

Endogenous Avidin Biotin

Endogenous biotin is present in the tissue such as kidney, liver, lymph node. Sequential 10 to 20 minutes incubation prior to staining protocol with 0.1% avidin followed by 0.01% biotin helps to quench the activity of endogenous avidin biotin.

Nonspecific Staining

Hydrophobic interaction is the most common cause of nonspecific background staining and is attachment of protein to connective tissue–collagen **(Fig. 7.26)**, squamous epithelium. Tissues that can affect are connective tissues, squamous epithelium, adipocytes.

Tissue proteins become hydrophobic during formalin fixation as the reactive amino acids are cross linked within and adjacent

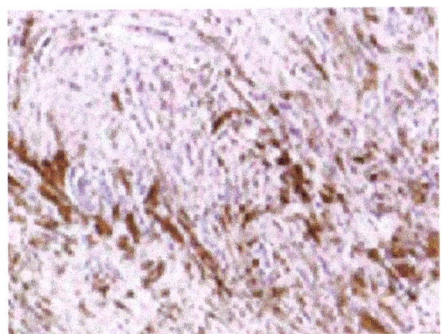

Fig. 7.26: Nonspecific staining of collagen.

proteins molecules. Hydrophobic cross linking can be affected by time (prolonged fixation), temperature and composition of fixative used. Hence the composition of fixative, fixation time, penetration capacity of fixative must be optimized and controlled.

Secondary antibodies can cause this type of background staining as being protein in nature. The antibody isoelectric point when closer to the pH of antibody diluent results in strong hydrophobic interaction causing background staining. Hence the ionic strength of antibody diluents has to be lowered. Isoelectric point (pI) is the pH at which a molecule carries no net electrical charge i.e., amphoteric in nature. Addition of proteins in blocking step and antibody diluents can be of help.

Treating with nonimmune serum for 10 minutes can reduce this effect. Protein blocking step must be carried just before application of primary antibody normal serum, bovine serum albumin, casein can be used for protein block **(Fig. 7.27)**

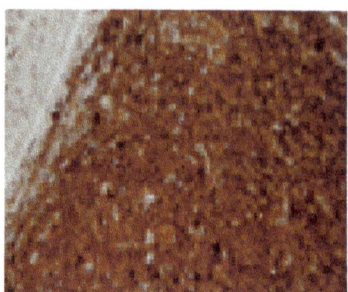

Fig. 7.27: Normal tonsil—heavy background due to ineffective protein block.

Antigen diffusion can result in spurious staining. This occurs when antigen may diffuse from its original site to the surrounding tissue.

This can result in because of
- Improper dilutions of antibodies
- Excessive epitope retrieval
- Drying of tissue before fixation

Other causes of nonspecific staining are:
- Improper washing of slides,
- Incomplete removal of paraffin form tissue sections.
- Poor penetration of tissue during fixation **(Fig. 7.28)**
- Folds in the tissue section, thick sections
- Storage conditions of reagents

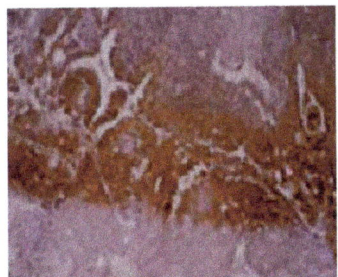

Fig. 7.28: Background due to poor penetration of fixative.

COMMON HITCHES OBSERVED AT END RESULT OF THE IMMUNOHISTOCHEMISTRY

False Negative Staining

Lack of staining OR weak staining in known positive tissues can result in because of

- Over fixation
- Precut control section not stored at correct temperature
- Control tissue is aged
- Improper selection of positive control
- Use of inadequate or incorrect antigen retrieval protocol
- Antibody concentration; storage conditions; date of expiry not monitored
- Incomplete deparaffinization
- Drying out of tissue section during staining
- Batch process failure.

False Positive Staining

Spurious staining can result because of excess or incorrect treatment on tissue sections. There may be cross reactivity of antibody with tissue section. Negative control plays a very important role in eliminating false positive staining.

- Excess of pretreatment can cause over digestion of tissue
- Inadequate tissue fixation
- Insufficient quenching of endogenous enzyme activity
- Unwanted antibody cross reactivity with the cells or cellular components
- Antibody concentration
- Improper washing

Weak or No Staining in Test Sample + Adequate Staining in Positive Control

Weak or no staining in test sample can result due to loss of antigenicity; repeat stain with different block

- Delayed fixation, autolyzed tissue, inadequate antigen retrieval
- Test sample and control tissue are not fixed or processed in identical manner
- Drying of test sample during staining

Uneven Staining in Test Sample

Inadequate primary fixation in formalin leading to secondary fixation with alcohol during processing

- Repeat test using different block
- Revalidate antigen retrieval process

APPLICATION OF IMMUNOHISTOCHEMISTRY

Immunohistochemistry has become an important ancillary test and is valuable in assessing tumor type and other features of prognostic and therapeutic importance. The technique also assists in refinement of diagnosis based on tissue morphology.

Majority of test request involve breast markers, panel for small cell undifferentiated carcinoma, metastatic carcinoma of unknown origin, markers for classification of lymphoma. In most of the carcinoma's presence or absence of metastases is an important prognostic indicator. Detection of the smallest metastatic deposit in lymph nodes is of help to the patient.

These are just guidelines on the basis of my experience, however the section of IHC markers for analysis is the responsibility of the pathologist.

Carcinoma of unknown origin denotes tumor in which primary site cannot be determined and their prognosis is poor. These tumors can be of lymphoid/epithelial/melanocytic/or mesenchyme origin.

Primary panel of antibodies **(Fig. 7.29)** suggested are, LCA (CD 45), cytokeratin AE1/AE3, S-100, SALL4, cytokeratin 7, cytokeratin 20.

Companion diagnostic markers—depending on primary panel additional makers specific to site are selected to run for final diagnosis.

A "Companion diagnostic" is a test for a predictive marker that classifies patient (tumors) into responders and no responders for a specific therapeutic agent companion diagnostics are designated as class III medical devices by the FDA, because the test equates directly in administration of drugs (Taylor 2014).

List of IHC markers—Her-2-Neu, C-kit, EGFR, Alk-1, PDL1 22c3, PDL1 28.2, PDL1(SP142) and upcoming more. Postanalytical phase involves opinion of the end user i.e., opinion of treating physician on test result. Performance of test is now directly related to medicine management as companion diagnostic test.

Optimizing Immunohistochemistry Protocol

- Tissue fixation and subsequent processing is most important factor causing poor immunostaining.

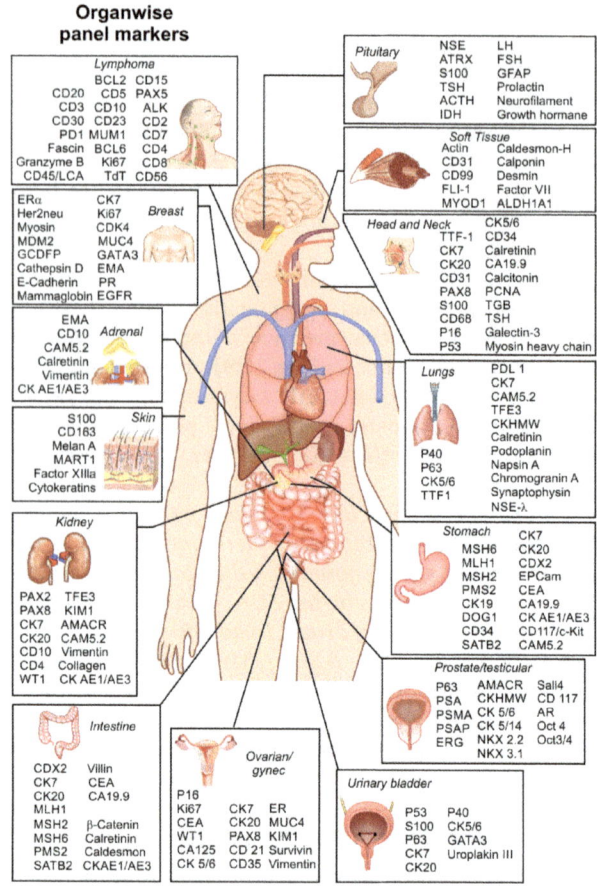

Fig. 7.29: Organwise panel marker.

For optimal tissue processing, the following conditions must be observed:
- Fixative should not be only readily available; it should also be in wide spread use to maximize the range and number of samples available for IHC studies.
- Prompt fixation of specimen is recommended.
- Fixation is best carried out close to neutral pH, in the range 6–8.
- The volume of the fixative should be 10:1 to the tissue.
- Cut thin slices of sections, 2 mm thick for better penetration.
- Fixation time should be optimized to avoid interference with antigen antibody reaction; should not exceed 24–48 hours.
- During embedding, the paraffin waxes >65°C must be avoided.
- Paraffin sections must be 3–4 µm thin. Sections are heated at 60°C for 1 hour or 37°C overnight.
- Do not use albuminized sides. Use poly-L-lysine coated slides.

❖ Washing is an important step in the staining. PH of washing buffer is maintained at 7.2 to 7.6; pH less or more than this value will result in improper staining.
- Slides are rinsed with buffer and are placed in buffer for 5 minutes x 2 to 3 changes.

❖ Antibody validation is mandatory step in immunostaining. Improper validation can result in either no staining or non-specific staining.
- pH of antibody diluent plays important role in maintaining antibody structure; if antibody deteriorates in diluent buffer can cause nonspecific staining.

❖ Expiry date, recommended storage for antibody, detection system conditions must be strictly monitored.

❖ Pipettes used for preparing antibodies must be calibrated at least once in the six months

IMMUNOFLUORESCENCE TECHNIQUE (IF)

The technique developed by Coons, Creech, Jones (1941).

The technique allowing visualization of specific antigen on tissue sections by binding a specific antibody conjugated with a fluorescent dye. Tissue sections are studied using fluorescence microscope.

The antibodies were labeled with fluorescent dye—fluorescein isocyanate (FITC).

FITC is commonly used dye in IF techniques. It has excitation and emission spectrum which covers the ultraviolet to blue light range and giving it apple green color.

Sir George G Stokes in 1852—coined the word Immunofluorescence.

August Kohler in 1904—invented fluorescent microscopy using UV light at very low wavelength.

M Haitinger in 1933—first developed staining with fluorescent dye on tissue sections.

Method

❖ Direct immunofluorescence
❖ Indirect immunofluorescence
 (*Refer to Labeling Methods*)

Application

❖ The technique is rapid and useful in early diagnosis of auto immune diseases in renal and skin diseases. IgG, IgM, IgA, C3, fibrinogen deposits in glomerulopathy. Similar deposits in skin

lesions, pemphigus, bullous pemphigoid, lichen planus, bullous SLE and other diseases.
- The observed results of immunofluorescence fades with the time hence needs to be stored in form of photographs.

Specimen

After biopsy, in institution, Tissue can be placed on the saline saturated gauze and transported to laboratory in a sealed container on ice or tissue is placed in Michel's transport medium and sent to laboratory.

List of antibodies for kidney and skin biopsy—IgG, IgM, IgA, C3, fibrinogen, C1q, κ and λ light chains (DAKO agilent)

Reagents

- Phosphate buffer saline (PBS) pH 7.4
- *Stock wash buffer*:

1 M Potassium citrate	32.44 g in 100 mL of distilled water
0.1 M Magnesium sulfate	2.46 g in 100 mL of distilled water
0.1 M N-ethylmaleimide	1.25 g in 100 mL of distilled water

- *Working wash buffer*:

1 M Potassium citrate	25 mL
0.1 M Magnesium sulfate	50 mL
0.1 M N-ethylmaleimide	50 mL
Distilled water	875 mL

  Adjust pH 7.0–7.2 using 1 N NaOH or 1 N HCl. Store at 4°C.

- *Transport medium: Michel's medium (pH 7.0–7.2)*

Ammonium sulfate	55 g
Working wash buffer	100 m

Add ammonium sulfate to working wash buffer. Mix well and store in dark plastic bottle at 4°C.

Note
1. N-ethylmaleimide works as anti autolytic agent. Handle carefully
2. Ammonium sulfate fixes tissue bound immunoglobulins without losing their antigenicity.
3. Transport medium at pH lower than 7.0–7.2 may cause variable results.
4. Specimens can be stored for 4–5 days in transport medium at room temperature.

Method

- Remove biopsy from transport medium in petri dish.
- Gross examines the tissue and document gross findings.
- Wash biopsy in the wash buffer solution to petri dish for 10 minutes × 3 changes.
- Remove biopsy using forcep; blot to remove excess wash buffer.
- Add cryo compound on chuck and freeze in cryostat.
- Trim cryo compund to obtain flat surface for the biopsy.
- Core can be placed straight or circular depending on the size of biopsy.
- Place chuck along with tissue back in cryostat.
- Once tissue is frozen trim very carefully at 10 μm till the tissue is completely exposed.
- Do fine cutting at 3–4 μm.
- Sections are picked up on coated slides and labeled with identification number immediately.
- Sections can be stored at –20°C till IF is done.

One section has to be immediately using rapid H&E stain.

Direct Immunofluorescence Staining (Fig. 7.30)

- Section is circled on the slide.
- Wash sections three times using wash buffer or PBS for 10 minutes each.
- Place slides in humid chamber and add primary antibody.
- Allow it incubate for 1 hour in dark.
- Wash slides in PBS for 10 minutes × 3 times
- Mount immediately with buffered glycerol using coverslips.
- Observe under fluorescence microscope.
- Store the slides at 4°C if delay for viewing in covered tray.

Indirect Immunofluorescence Staining

- Wash sections in PBS for 10 minutes × 3 times.
- Add primary antibody to the section (prediluted or optimally titrated).
- Incubate in dark for 1 hour.
- Wash in buffer 10 minutes × 3 times
- Add secondary to the slide and incubate for 30 minutes in dark.
- Wash in buffer 10 minutes × 3 times
- Mount immediately with buffered glycerol using coverslips.

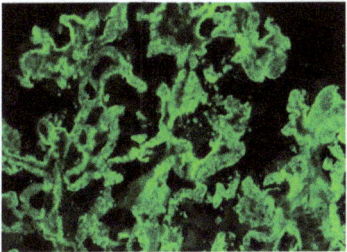

Fig. 7.30: Direct immunofluorescence—C3 renal biopsy.

IN SITU HYBRIDIZATION (ISH)

The technique is used for precise detection and localization of a specific nucleic acid sequence within a histologic section. The basic principle of ISH is that the nucleic acids within a histologic specimen can be detected by the hybridization of a complementary nucleic acid probe in which a reporter molecule is attached. Common nonradioactive labels for probe are fluorescein and digoxigenin. Subsequent visualization of the reporter molecule localizes DNA or RNA sequences in tissue or cells samples. The technique has evolved detection of the probe targeted hybrid using the principle of immunohistochemistry.

This method includes incubation with a mouse anti- fluorescein or digoxigenin antibody, followed by secondary antibody HRP conjugate with. After addition of an appropriate substrate for the enzyme (such as DAB—diaminobenzidine-solution), a colored reaction product (brown) is observed at the location of the probe-target hybrid. Microscopic examination of the slide provides visual interpretation of the staining results. Subsequent washing steps remove any probe that is not bound or that is nonspecifically bound to the tissue section.

Reagents

- Supersensitive one-step polymer HRP ISH detection system
- Positively charged slides
- Positive control
- Negative control
- Dehydration and clearing solutions

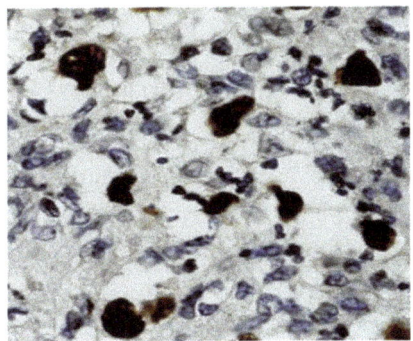

Fig. 7.31: EBER positive.

Preparation of DAB—mix 2 drops (80 μL) of DAB chromogen with 1 mL of substrate buffer. Always prepare fresh before use.

Specimen

Formalin fixed paraffin embedded blocks of selected specimen.

Quality Control

Each test run must include both positive and negative control which help us to confirm the test performance.

Positive control probe: The positive probe is known to be complementary to nucleic acid sequences in a test tissue slide that is processed in a manner identical to the slides that are being tested.

Negative control probe: A negative probe is known not to be complementary to the target nucleic acid sequences that are being detected.

Standard Staining Protocol

- Xylene — 3 changes × 5 minutes each
- Ethanol — 2 changes × 5 minutes each
- Wash in running water — 5 minutes
- Wash in distilled water — 2 minutes
- Hydrogen peroxide — 10 minutes
- Buffer wash — 2 changes × 3 minutes each
- Pepsin — 10 minutes
- Buffer wash — 2 minutes
- 10% formaldehyde — 10 minutes
- Buffer wash — 2 changes × 3 minutes each.
- Apply EBER probe (**Fig. 7.31**) and cover slip and then seal the edges with fevibond.
- Keep the slides in hybridizer -1programme (85°C) for 5 minutes (*refer* to probe data sheet)
- Remove slides and keep in humidity chamber at 37°C in the incubator overnight.

Next Day

- Remove the cover slip and wash with buffer — 3 changes × 5 minutes each
- Keep in wash buffer — 10 minutes
- Power block — 10 minutes
- Do not wash, just wipe excess power block.
- Add anti-probe fluorescent antibody and incubate at 37°C for 30 minutes
- Buffer wash — 2 changes × 3 minutes each
- Apply HRP and incubate at room temperature for 30 minutes.
- Buffer wash — 2 changes × 5 minutes each
- Apply DAB reagent — 5–10 minutes

- Buffer wash — 2 changes × 5 minutes each
- Counter stain with hematoxylin — 4–8 minutes
- Add buffer and keep for bluing — 10 minutes
- Wash with fresh buffer — 5 minutes
- Wash with running water — 5 minutes
- Dehydrate clear and mount.

Result

Positive: Brown color specific to nucleus.

Note

- Thin uniform sections on positively charged slides.
- Deparaffinization and clearing steps needs to be monitored.
- Mayer's Hematoxyline is preferred to use as progressive type.
- Wash Solution steps are specific to a probe. Always refer to probe data sheet.
- Antigen retrieval protocol is specific to probe. Always check to probe data sheet for antigen retrieval protocol.
- Any probe used with this method need to have fluorescein molecule attached with it.
- Use disposable gloves during staining protocol.

REFERENCE

Biogenex ISH kit protocol for EBER.

BIBLIOGRAPHY

1. Bancroft JD and Stevens A. Theory and practice of histological techniques. 8th edition.
2. Battifora H, Koppinsky IM, J HistochemCytochem. 1986;34:1095-1100.

3. Battifora H. Assessment of antigen damage in immunohistochemistry. The Vimentin internal control: Am J Clin. Pathol.1991;96:669.
4. Biogenex ISH kit protocol for EBER.
5. Clive R Taylor. Predictive biomarkers and companion diagnostics. The future of immunohistochemistry - `in situ proteomics `or just a `stain'?; Appl Immunohistochem Mol Morphol. 2014(September);22(8): 555-561.
6. David J Dabbs. Diagnostic immunohistochemistry. 5th edition.
7. Embedded tissue sections by pressure cooking: a comparison with microwave heating and traditional methods. Advances in anatomic pathology. 1995;2(1): 60-64.
8. Immunohistochemical Staining Methods, 6th edition. DAKO.
9. J. Auld. Antigen unmasking in routinely processed paraffin sections by pressure cooking.
10. K Miller, J Auld, et. al. Antigen unmasking in formalin fixed routinely processed paraffin wax.
11. Koss's Diagnostic cytology, 5th edition.
12. Larry J Fowler, MD; Whitney A. Lachar, MD. Application of Immunohistochemistry to cytology. Arch Pathol Lab Med. 2008;132:373-383.
13. Leong ASY, Gilham PN. The effects of progressive formaldehyde fixation on the tissue antigen. Pathol. 1989;21:266.
14. Rodney T Miller. Technical immunohistochemistry. Achieving reliability and reproducibility of immunostains. MD.
15. Shi S-R, Cote RJ, Chaiwun B, Young LL, Shi Y, Hawes D, et. al. Standardization of imunohistochemistry based on antigen retrieval technique for routine formalin-fixed tissue sections. Appl Immunohistochem.1998;6:89-96.
16. Shi S-R, Cote RJ, Taylor CR. J HistochemCytochem. 1997;45(3):327-343.
17. Taylor and Cote. A diagnostic tool for surgical pathologist.
18. UK NEQUAS IMMUNOCYTCHEM. news spring. 1994;(3).

Annexures

ANNEXURE I

Histopathology, cytology, immunohistochemistry pure water is plays important role for preparing stain, reagents and buffers.

Distilled Water

Distilled water is produced by a process of distillation. Distillation involves boiling of water and condensing vapor into clean container leaving solid contaminants behind. Thus, distillation produces very pure water. Distilled water must be stored in sterile containers for laboratory use.

Deionized Water

Economic solution for pure water. Deionized water is water that has had all ions removed. Deionization focuses on contaminants that carry an electric charge, which are mineral ions. Purification technologies that are used for deionization are electrodeionization (EDI), ion exchange (XI), deionization with reverse osmosis resulting in formation of pure water. Deionized water is used as routine in all laboratory divisions

RO Water—Reverse Osmosis Water

Uses a semipermeable membrane to remove ions, molecules, and larger particles from water.

Osmosis is a natural process. When two solutions with different concentrations of a solute are separated by a semipermeable membrane, the solvent has a tendency to move from low to high solute concentrations till equilibrium.

Reverse osmosis can remove many types of dissolved and suspended species from water, including bacteria and is used in both industrial processes and the production of potable water.

ANNEXURE II

Preparation of Solutions

Solution by definition is a homogenous mixture of two or more substances in relative amounts that can be varied continuously up to what is called limit of solubility.

Different Solutions

- *Normal saline:* 0.9% of Sodium chloride.
- *Percentage solution:* The solution expressed in the unit %. It may be % by weight -w/v or % by volume v/v.

For example,

Preparation of w/v solutions		Prepare 500 mL of 15% nitric acid (v/v)
1%	1g dissolved in 100 mL of solvent	15% = 15 mL nitric acid in 85 mL of water
5%	5 g dissolved in 100 mL of solvent	To prepare 500 mL of 15% is 15 x 5 = 75 mL; 500 mL –75 mL = 425 mL = to add 75 mL of nitric acid in 425 mL of water

Preparation of v/v solutions	
5%	5 mL of solute in 95 mL of water
1%	1 mL of solute in 99 mL of water
0.1%	10 mL of 1% in 90 mL of water
0.01%	1 mL of 1% in 99 mL of water
0.001%	1 mL of 0.1% in 99 mL of water

❖ **Normal solution and molar solution**

Most of the reagents have formula weight are listed on the reagent bottle.

Normality is defined as the gram equivalent of the solute dissolved per liter of the solution. Normality is expressed as N. Molarity is defined as the gram molecular weight dissolved per litre of the solution. Molarity is expressed as M.

For example:
- Molecular weight of NaCl 58.44 (atomic weight of Na 22.99, Cl 35.45)
- To prepare 1 M NaCl 58.44 g of NaCl to be dissolved in 1000 mL of distilled water.
- To calculate molecular weight and equivalent weight of H_2SO_4–
  Atomic weight of H 1.008, S 32.06, O 16
  Molecular weight = $2(1/008) + 32.06 + 4(16) = 98.08$ g/mol
  Equivalent weight = molecular weight/number of replaceable hydrogen
  Therefore, equivalent weight of H_2SO_4 is $98.08/2 = 49.04$

❖ **Saturated solution:** A solution that contains a maximum amount of a particular solute that will dissolve at desired temperature.

❖ **Hydrates:** It is very important to distinguish between the terms anhydrous and hydrous. If a compound is hydrated it contains water in close chemical union and number of water molecules are specified. Anhydrous is crystalline compound with No water content.

❖ **Buffer solution**

A buffer solution is one which resists changes in pH when small quantities of an acid or alkali are added to it.

- *When base is added to buffer solution:* The hydrogen ions from the acidic component combine with hydroxyl ions from the base and water is formed. Hence no significant change in the pH of the buffer will take place.
- *When acid is added to a buffer solution:* The excess hydrogen ions from the added acid are removed by the salt ions to form more molecules of the unionized weak acid. Hence again no significant change in the pH of the buffer will take place.

Index

Page numbers followed by *f* refer to figure and *t* refer to table

A

Absolute isopropyl alcohol 203, 204
Acetaldehyde 191
Acetic acid 184, 189
Acetone 184, 191, 194
Acid
    alcohol 251
    dyes 247
Acinetobacter anitratus 156
Acrolein 192
Additive 184
Adenovirus 156
Adequate fixative, use of 181
Adsorption 248
Advancement hand wheel 220
Affinity 266
Agitation 195
Agrobacterium tumefaciens 25
Air filtration system 173
Alcohol 184, 189, 193, 261
Alcoholic ammonia solution 252
Alkaline phosphatase 274, 319
    anti alkaline phosphatase method 275*f*
    conjugated polymer 318
Allele-specific probes 30
Alpha-fetoprotein 321*f*
Alum hematoxylin 251, 253
Aluminum sulfate 255
Amino acids 266
Ammonium sulfate 333
Amplichain 100, 122, 123, 125
    chikungunya 127, 140
        kit 142*t*, 157, 158
        reagents 145
        uses TaqMan 141
    cytomegalovirus 127
    dengue 127
    Ex 32 103, 120, 127, 136
        operating instructions for 105
    human leukocyte antigens-B27 127
    human papillomavirus infection 16 and 18 127
    instrument 103
    malaria 127
    monotest 104
    multitest 104
    mycobacterium tuberculosis 127
        polymerase chain reaction reagent 113*f*

polymerase chain reaction station 103
quantitative polymerase chain reaction station 103, 111, 112, 112f, 120
   instrument 150
   login window 115f
   test run, set of 115
reagents 121, 126
universal 130, 136, 137, 146
   kit 107, 130
   lysis 132
   plate 136
   prefilled cartridges 110, 110f
   specificity of 137

Amplification 59, 68, 150
   continued rounds of 91
   experiment 42
   reaction 52
   temperature of 152t
   time of 152t
Amplified deoxyribonucleic acid 77
AmpliTaq deoxyribonucleic acid polymerase 78
Amplitude, high 65, 66f
Analyte specific reagent 303
Analytical sensitivity 157
Analytical specificity 137, 155
   using polymerase chain reaction 137t
Anaplastic lymphoma kinase 6
Ancient deoxyribonucleic acid, amplification of 97
Ancillary tests 163, 166
Animal cells 25
Annealing 35, 87
   temperature 89
Anthraquinone dyes 245
Anti roll guide plate 236
Anti-alkaline phosphatase 274

Antibody 267, 279, 303
   basic monomer unit of 267
   concentrated 301, 310, 328
   description 302
   improper dilutions of 326
   ready to use 301
   secondary 273, 325
   selection of 267
   structure of 268f
   validation 285, 300
   Y molecule of 267
Antigen 266
   antibody reaction 266, 312
   retrieval 289, 290f
      heat pretreatment for 265
      method 285
      protocols 267
      solution 302
   specific 267
Apathy's medium 242
   Highman's modification of 242
Apocrine sweat glands, epithelium of 305
Appropriate acids, use of 238
Argentaffin 248
Argyrophil 248
Artificial intelligence, role of 21
Arylmethane dyes 245
Ascitic fluid 272
Aspirates 163
Autolysis 178
Automated labeling system 168
Automated nucleic acid extraction system 128
Automatic coverslipper 241f
Automatic knife sharpener 222, 223f
Automation 265
   types of 258
Autostainers, types of 319
Auxochrome 244, 246

Avidin-biotin 265
  complex method 275, 276f
Axillary tail 176f
Azine 245
Azo group 245

B

B lymphocytes 266
Bacillus subtilis 137, 156
Bacteria 25
Bacterial cells 25
Bactofection 25
Bar code 168f
Base sledge microtome 218
Basic dyes 247
Batch process failure 327
Battifora 306
Benzene 194
  ring compound 244
Beta coronavirus, test for 161
Beta-actin 58
Big resection specimens 174
Biliary tract 305
Biliary tree, carcinomas of 305
Binding, strength of 266
Biopsy
  endoscopic 213
  excision 165
  punch needle with plunger 309f
  remove 334
Biosafety cabinet 143
Biotechnology company 76
Biotin 89, 280
Bird flu 15
Blocks
  holder 220
  selection of 304, 305t
Blotting 26
  paper 228
Bluing 251, 257
  solutions 252
Blunt blade 231
Blunt knife 231
Body fluids 163
Bone marrow 213
  biopsy, fixation of 188
  multiple bits 213f
Bony specimens 174
Bouin's fluid 190
Bovine serum albumin 325
Breast
  tissue 176f
  tumor 174f
Buffer 41, 306
  large volume of 295
  preparation of 299
  solution 344
    pH of 293
  wash 338, 339
Buffered formal 188, 191
  sucrose 189

C

Calf alkaline phosphatase 280
Calibrator graph 72, 72f
Cancer 9, 73, 86
Candida albicans 137, 156
Capillary gap 320
  technique 320
Carbohydrates 164
Carbon 245
Carcinoma 305, 329
  hepatocellular 321f
Carney's fixative 187
Carousel type tissue processors 197, 199f
Catalyzed reporter deposition techniques 265

Index

Catalyzed signal amplification method 276
Celestine blue-alum hematoxylin method 256
Cell
    block, preparation of 317
    line controls 306
    lysis 44
    macromolecules of 164
    molecular components of 5
Cellular processes 73
Cellular, enzymatic destruction of 179
Centrifugation 45
Cepheid 99
Cervix 166
Cesium chloride 42
Chaotropic salt solution 44
Charged polypeptides 294
Chemical 238
    oxidation 250
Chikungunya 153, 154, 156
    ribonucleic acid, qualitative detection of 154
    test for 160
    virus 137, 140
        ribonucleic acid of 140
Chlamydia trachomatis, test for 160
Chloral hydrate 254
Chloroform 194
Cholera, test for 161
Chromic acid 184
Chromium potassium sulfate 226
Chromogen 244, 245, 280
    substrate 318
Chromogranin S 323
Chromophore group 245
Chromyl chloride 192
Circular deoxyribonucleic acid microarrays 32
Citrate buffer 300

Citric acid 254
Clinical sample integrity 82
Clostridium difficile, test for 161
Coagulant fixative 184
Coarse hand wheel 219, 220
Cold plate 209
Collagen, nonspecific staining of 325*f*
Colloidal gold labels 280
Column separation 45
Community health centre 103, 122
Compatible real-time polymerase chain reaction instruments 151
Complementary nucleotides 90
Complete
    process control 126
    resection 166
Component 131, 142, 147-149
Concentration 181
Condensing vapor 341
Cone biopsy 166
Conventional prenatal tests 73
Cooling blocks 143
Copper sulfate 281
Correlation coefficient 50, 50*f*
Cost-effective molecular test system 102
Counter stain 248, 339
Covalent bonding 243, 247
COVID-19 162
    pandemic 1
    test for 161, 162
Cross-sample contamination 83
Cryostat 233
    cut sections 191
    disinfection 233
    functional view 234*f*
    support 234
    temperature 233
Crystalline compound 344
Cupric salts 184
Cut specimens 173

Cycle threshold 41
Cyclophilin A 58
Cystic fibrosis 23
Cytology 341
Cytomegalovirus 156
   test for 161
Cytoplasm 247, 323
Cytoskeletal gene 58

D

Deep well plate 108*f*
Degraded reagents 63
Dehydration 164*f*, 179, 193, 193*f*, 257, 261, 336
   stage 216
Deionized water 341, 342
Delafield's hematoxylin 254
Denaturation 87, 89
Dengue
   test for 160, 162
   virus 137
Dense peritumoral lymphocytic inflammation 10*f*
Deoxyribonucleic acid 5, 73, 90
   analysis of 22
   barcoding, utilization of 74
   based phylogenies, construction of 97
   chips 33
   cloning application 97
   copy-number alterations 11
   deletions of 7
   extraction kit, components of 131*t*
   microarray 32, 33*f*, 74
   molecules 34
   nonspecific amplification of 98
   polymerase 37, 38*f*, 77, 87
      epsilon 11
      use of 76
   profiling 97
   segments 77
   sequences 24, 32, 76
Deoxyribonucleotide triphosphate 39, 87
Deparaffinization 239, 257, 286
Detection system 276*f*, 285, 302
Diaminobenzidine 264, 280
   solution 336
Dibasic sodium phosphate anhydrous 300
Dibutylphthalate 243
Digital images 174
Digital pathology 18
   clinical deployment of 18
Digoxigenin 336
Direct immunofluorescence staining 332, 335, 335*f*
Direct labeling method 273*f*
Disposable blades 224*f*, 226
Disposable nuclease-free plasticware 133
Dissociation curve 55
Distilled water 254, 255, 341
Distorted graph 69, 69*f*
Dithionite 216
Domestic microwave oven pretreatment 295
Double stain block 318
Double-stranded deoxyribonucleotide 36, 55
Drain excess water 229
Drug development 74
Drying 239, 286
   artifacts 237
Dye 238, 244, 245
   aggregation 247
   binding, action for 246
   classification of 245, 247
   formation of 244
   selection 249

Index

E

Ebola 15
Effective amplification, important for 98
Ehrlich's hematoxylin 255
Electrodeionization 341
Electrophoresis 29, 35
Elution buffer 135
Embedding 163
    cassette 211
    images 213f
    molds 208
    station 210f
Emergency pullout eye washer 173
Enclosed tissue processor 199, 200f
Endocervix, epithelial cells of 305
Endogenous alkaline phosphatase 324
Endogenous avidin biotin 324
Endogenous enzyme activity 323
Endogenous peroxidase 323
Endometrial carcinoma 9
    molecular subgroup of 10f, 13, 13t, 14
Endometrioid 9
Endometrium 305
Endoscope 166
Enterobacter cloacae 156
Enterococcus faecalis 137, 156
Enzymatic method 45
Enzyme 80
    amounts of 41
    digestion 265, 291, 292
        length of 292
    horseradish peroxidase, development of 264
    labels 279
    pretreatment 292
    quality 52
    substrate reaction, results of 280
Eosin-phloxine solution 251

Epidermal growth factor receptor gene 6
Epithelioid sarcoma 305
Epstein-Barr virus 156
Escherichia coli 137, 156
Ethanol 132, 216, 338
    formalin 317
    volume of 107, 134
Ethidium bromide 42
Ethyl alcohol 187, 194
Ethylene glycol 255, 256
Eukaryotic cell 25, 26
Excessive epitope retrieval 326
Exponential rate 90
Extension 35, 87, 89
Extracellular molecules 179
Extraction hose, adapter piece for 235

F

Fallopian tube 305
Ferric ammonium sulfate 256
Fetus 305
Fibrinogen deposits 332
Fingerprints 33
Fixation 179, 164, 183
    duration of 291
    using perfusion 183
Fixative 179, 183, 331
    adequate amount of 182f
    histochemical 184, 191
    poor penetration of 327f
    preparation of 188
    volume ratio of 182, 182f
Floaters 215
Fluorescence 336
    chemistries 61
    dye 332
        based real-time polymerase chain reaction 55f
    in situ hybridization 29, 30f

isocyanate 332
isothiocyanate 279
labelled oligonucleotide probes 29
labels 279
microscopy 31
probe 40
signal 152
    change in 46
Fluoroquinolone resistant mycobacterium tuberculosis, test for 161
Forceps 210
Formal saline 202, 203
Formaldehyde 184, 185, 188, 191
    fixation 285f
Formalin 188, 189
    fixation, mechanism of 185
    fixed paraffin embedded tissue blocks 177, 263
    fumes, backdraft extraction of 173
    jar 215
Freeze drying technique 184
Freezing microtome 218
Fresh tissue, cryostat cut sections of 191
Frozen section 163, 231
    accuracy 237
    applications of 231
    staining for 236
Fructose syrup 242

G

Gallbladder 166
Gardnerella vaginalis 156
Gauze piece 211
Gel electrophoresis 29
Gelatin 226
Gendre's solution 190
Gene
    cloning 97
    functional analysis of 97
    mutagenesis 97
    rearrangements 24
    specific primers 37
Genetic
    disease 4, 86
    fingerprints, analysis of 97
GeneXpert 99
Genomic 6
Genotypes, differentiation of 97
Geographical diversity 81
Gill's hematoxylin 255
Glacial acetic acid 188, 255
Glass slides 288
Glomerulopathy 332
Glutaraldehyde 184, 187, 192
    phosphate dehydrogenase 58
Glycerin 242, 256
Glycerol 216, 226
Glycogen 187
Glycolysis pathway 58
Glyoxal 184
Group B streptococcus 161
Gynecological malignancy 9

H

H and E staining, automation for 258, 259f
H1N1 15
    test for 160
H3N2, test for 160
Haematoxylin 255
Haemophilus influenzae type B, test for 162
Handling core biopsy 175f
Hanker-Yate's reagent 280
Harri's hematoxylin 254, 257
Hazy sections 261
Heat 184, 195
    denaturation 90
    mediated antigen retrieval 293
    retrieval method 302

Heating
    and bubbling technology 199, 204
    time and temperature 293, 294f
Heiffor knife 221
Helly's fluid 190
Hematologic disease 4
Hematoxylin 244, 249, 255, 339
    and eosin stain 249
        slides 258f
    types of 252
Hemochromatosis 23
Hepatitis
    A virus, test for 160
    B virus 137, 156
        test for 160
    C virus 137, 156
        test for 160
    E virus, test for 160
Herpes simplex virus 156
    test for 161
High background noise graph 67, 67f
Histopathology 163, 341
    specimen 165
Homogenous mixture 342
Horseradish peroxidase 273, 279, 319
    catalytic activity of 276
    complex 277
Hot
    air oven 195, 227
    plate 227
Human brain 19
Human immunodeficiency virus 137, 156
    test for 160
Human leukocyte antigens-B27 137
    detection of 127
    test for 161
Human papillomavirus 156
    high risk types, test for 161
Human specimen 147
    negative extraction control 149

Human whole blood 154
Humidity chamber 292
Hybridization 35
Hybridoma techniques, development of 265
Hydrates 344
Hydration 286
    preparation of 239
Hydrogen
    bonding 243, 246
    ions 344
    peroxide 338
Hydrophobia 289
Hydrophobic
    attractive forces 294
    binding 247
    interaction 243, 324

I

Ice crystals 237
Ideal calibrator graph 71, 71f
Ideal immunostaining, hallmarks of 320
Immunofluorescence 279
    technique 264, 332
Immunohistochemistry 163, 178, 263, 267, 316, 327, 328
    applications of 328
    automation in 319
    markers 329
    multiple staining in 318
    preparation 321
    pure water 341
    staining 282
        kit 287f
In situ hybridization 336
Inadequate tissue fixation 328
Incision biopsy 165
Incomplete decalcification tissues 207
Incomplete impregnation process 230
Inconsistent spacing 72, 72f

Incubator 132
Indirect immunofluorescence 332
  staining 335
Indirect labeling method 274f
Infectious disease 4, 23, 73
Influenza
  A virus, test for 161, 162
  B virus, test for 161, 162
Inherited genetic diseases 23
Inhibitors, presence of 63, 65, 67, 72
Instrument software 69, 70
Instrumentation 61, 127
Interferometer 31
Invalid graph 63, 63f
Ion exchange 341
Ionic binding 246
Ionophoresis 29
Iron hematoxylin 252, 253
Isoniazid resistant mycobacterium
    tuberculosis, test for 160
Isopropanol 43
Isopropyl alcohol 194, 195, 202, 203,
    204, 205, 257
Isotope 303

J

Japanese encephalitis virus, test for 162

K

Kidney, antibody for 333
Kit
  components 130, 141
  liquid components of 143
Knife
  guard 235
  holder 219, 220
  sharpening 222
Kyasanur forest disease, test for 162

L

Labeled streptavidin-biotin method 276
Laboratory
  decentralization of 82
  developed tests 18
  information system 168
Lead hematoxylin 252
Legionella 137, 156
Leica bond max 320
Leishmaniasis, test for 162
Leptospira, test for 161
Leukemia 86
Leukhartz mold 208
Leukocyte antigen typing 23
Linear type 259
Lipids 164, 266
Liquid cover slip method 320
Lithium carbonate solution 252
Loading deep well plate 107
Lock hand wheel 236
Locked nucleic acid, detection of 27
Log-linear phase, slope of 52, 53f
Low amplitude 65, 65f
Low infrastructure setup 102
Lumpectomy specimens 166
Lymph nodes 166, 329
Lymphoid tissue 188
Lymphomas 86
Lyophilized reagents, reconstitution of
    146, 148
Lyophilized single tube polymerase
    chain reaction mix 81

M

Macromolecule blotting 26
Macromolecules, major 164
Macroscopic examination 163

Index

Magnesium
    concentration 39
    sulfate 333
Magnetic beads
    based single kit 126
    method 44, 45f, 130, 134
Magnetic stand 129, 132, 135
Mammary gland 305
Manual hematoxylin and eosin staining protocol 257
Manual nucleic acid extraction 128
Manual rotary microtome 219
Manufacturer's recommendations sheet 302
Martius scarlet blue method 256
Master mix 41, 147, 147t, 148t
Maternal plasma 73
Mayer's egg albumin 226
Mayer's hematoxylin 253
Measles virus, test for 162
Melting curve 55
Melting point 55
Membrane 213f
Mercuric chloride 184, 186, 189, 190
    pigment 190
Mesothelial cells 305
Metachromatic dye 248
Metachromatic stain 236
Metachrome 248
Metal 220
    holder 207f
    probe 170
Metaphase 30
Methicillin resistant Staphylococcus aureus, test for 161
Method selection criteria 318
Methylation-specific polymerase chain reaction 96
Michel's medium 333

Micro polymer
    detection kits 319
    technology 319
Microarray 32
    reader 32
    technology 74
Micropipettes 132
    range of 310
Microsatellite instability 11
Microscopic examination 163
Microtome 217f
    attachment, holders for 209f
    care of 229
    important features of 219
    knives 220
        maintenance of 223
    maintenance of 229
    parts of 219
Microtomy 163, 165, 216
    knife angle for 224, 225f
Microwave
    based tissue processor 201f, 205
    fixation 184
    oven 294, 295f
Mismatch repair proteins 10f
Molar solution 343
Molecular biology 1, 22
    field of 23
Molecular cloning 24, 25f
Molecular diagnostics 22, 23, 73, 79, 124
    applications of 73
    techniques 23, 24
        applications of 73
    tests 15, 82
Molecular imaging 21
Molecular pathology 1, 4, 6, 8, 9, 15, 20
    association for 23
    clinical specialties of 2f
    laboratories 34
    techniques of 3f

Molecular technique 34
Molecular testing 103
Molybdenum hematoxylin 252
Monkeypox virus, test for 162
Monobasic potassium phosphate anhydrous 300
Monoclonal antibody 270, 270f, 272
    production of 271f
Mordant dyes 248
Mounting 165, 239, 287
    medium, types of 241
Mucormycosis, test for 162
Multiple dyes 56
Multiple extraction reagents 124
Multiple genes, expression rate of 32
Multiple markers, simultaneous visualization of 318
Multitumor paraffin blocks, use of 308
Multitumor tissue block 308f, 310
Mumps virus, test for 162
Muscle tissue 213
Mutation 15
Mycobacteria, nontuberculous 161
Mycobacterium
    leprae, test for 162
    tuberculosis 137
        bacteria 127
        complex 102
        test for 160-162
Mycoplasma genitalium, test for 162

N

Natural dyes 244
Natural resinous medium 243
Negative extraction control 143, 147, 153t
Neisseria gonorrhoeae, test for 160, 162
N-ethylmaleimide works 334
Neurotrophic receptor tyrosine kinase 6
Neutral buffered formalin 177

Neutral dyes 248
New antibody, validation of 312, 312t
Next-generation sequencing 6
Nipah virus 15
    test for 161
Nitrogen 245
No template control 57, 149
    table of 153t
Nonadditive 184
Noncoagulant fixative 184, 185
Nonoptimal reagent concentrations, use of 52
Normal saline 342
Northern blotting 26, 27f, 262
    technique, major disadvantages of 27
Nuclear features, high-grade 10f
Nuclease 144
    free
        microtips 132
        water 40, 148
    inactivating agents 132
Nucleic acid 80, 114, 164, 266
    adsorption 44, 140
    based testing, applications of 22
    extraction 15, 42, 127, 136, 146
        fully automated 105f
        techniques 42
    handling area 150
    testing automation 15
Nucleotides 39
    sequences, examination of 22

O

Oligonucleotide 33, 35, 40
    sequences 33
    set of 40
    specific 94
Onchrome 248
Oncology 23

Open tissue processor 197, 198f
Optimum temperature, use of 237
Organwise panel marker 330f
Origin, primary site of 33
Oscillation rate 203
Osmium tetraoxide 188
Osmolality 182
Osmosis 342
Ovarian sex cord tumors 305
Overnight protocol 203, 204
Oxazine dyes 245
Oxidation, natural 250
Oxygen 245

P

P53 tumor suppressor gene 30
Pancreas 305
Paraffin
    block 230
        holder 208
    sections 225, 331
    wax 165, 194, 195, 202-205, 210, 212, 213
        bath, temperature of 215
Parameter polymerase chain reaction testing 160
Parasitic pathogens 86
Patchy staining 261
Pathology, role of 1
Pathophysiological information 21
Pelvic peritoneum, small round cell tumor of 305
Penetration 185
Pepsin 292, 338
Peptides 266
Peritoneal cavity 272
Peroxidase
    anti peroxidase
        method 274, 275f
        technique 265
    conjugated polymer 318
Personal protective equipment accessories 145
pH
    changes in 344
    levels 187
Phenol-chloroform
    extraction 42
    solution, mixing of 42
Phosphate buffer
    pH 292
    saline 300, 333
Phthalocyanine 245
Picric acid 184, 187, 190
Place multiple tissue fragments 213
Plasmid 25, 25f, 157
Plasmodium
    falciparum, test for 160
    vivax, test for 160
Polyclonal antibody 267, 268, 269f, 278f
Poly-L-lysine coated slides, preparation of 288
Polymer based
    detection systems 306
    techniques 277
Polymerase
    chain reaction 15, 34, 35f, 77, 85, 88f, 97, 100
        amplification 92
        applications of 97
        asymmetric 96
        based technology 145
        components 37
        cycle 46f
        detection, molecular beacon based 94f
        diagnostic technology 85
        evolution of 75, 85
        hood 143

ligation-mediated 96
master mix 41
multiplex 7, 34, 59, 60f, 96
nested 91, 96
over conventional techniques, advantages of 97
powerful amplification of 99
principle of 87, 100
products, analysis of 76
reagents 98, 114
technique 77, 97
testing 99, 131t
tube 113f-115f, 118f, 143
types of 91
working area requirements 145
enzymes, normal 89
heat-resistant 34
Polymerization 35
Polymorphism 15
Polypeptide chains, prevent intertwining of 294
Polysaccharides 266
Polyvinylidene fluoride 28
Poor tissue fixation 178
Positive control probe 337
Positive sense single-stranded genome 140
Post staining procedures 239, 287
Potassium
alum 255
citrate 333
dichromate 184, 186, 189, 190
Pragmatic molecular classifiers 12
Preanalytical phase 282, 283
Predictive markers, validation of 313
Predictive molecular pathology, emergence of 1
Prefilled individual test cartridge 136

Prefilled plate 136
Prenatal tests 73
Pressure cooker 296, 297f
pretreatment 296
Primary antibody 273, 274, 301, 302, 318
selection of 285
staining pattern of 323f
validation of 285, 300, 310
Primary reaction 91
Probe labelling, combination of 31
Programmable pressure cooker, pretreatment of 297
Propylene oxide 194
Protective equipment accessories 145
Protein 164
adhesives 226
blocking 325
deoxyribonucleic acid hybridizations 26
ionized amino groups of 247
protein interactions 26
Proto-oncogene 1 6
Pseudomonas aeruginosa 137, 156
test for 162
PT module 298, 298f
Punch biopsy 166
Pure water, economic solution for 341
Purification 101
Putrefaction 178

Q

Qiagen 151
Q-positive segment 32
Quality control 153, 261, 317, 337
Quality improvement criteria 285
Quantitative analysis 28
Quantitative polymerase chain reaction instrument, result window of 119f

Quantitative reverse transcriptase polymerase chain reaction 37
Quick freezer shelf 235

R

Rabbit monoclonal antibodies, production of 266
Rabies virus, test for 161
Random primers 37
Rapid fixation 190
Reagent 107, 134, 134t, 253, 288, 333, 336
    handling of 63, 72, 82
    kit contains reagents 130
    preparation of 134
    sensitivity 124
    storage 124
        conditions of 326
    tissue interaction 246
Real-time polymerase chain reaction 92, 140
    advantages of 36
    analysis 45
    fluorescence detection systems 55
    kits 127, 140
    plot, depiction of 92f
    system 100
    TaqMan probe-based principle 104
Receptor tyrosine kinase 6
Refractive index 242
Rehydration 164, 257
Requisition form 169
Respiratory syncytial virus, test for 162
Restriction fragment length polymorphisms 15
Reverse osmosis 341, 342
Reverse osmosis water 342
Reverse transcriptase-polymerase chain reaction 91
    journey of 80

Ribonucleic acid 5, 140
    extraction kit, components of 131t
    sequencing 22
    virus 140
Ribosomal subunit 58
Rifampicin resistant mycobacterium tuberculosis, test for 160
Robotic arm 259
Rocking microtome 217, 218
Rotary microtome 217-219
    fully automated 219
Rotavirus, test for 162
Rubella virus, test for 162
Running Amplichain Universal Kit 107
Running test 116
    parameter 110
Rush biopsy protocol 203, 204

S

Salmonella 161
    enterica 137, 156
Scalpel 228
    blades 170
Scott's tap water 252
Scrub typhus, test for 161
Semi-automated rotary microtome 219
Semipermeable membrane 342
Sensitivity 158, 164, 301
    direct measure of 51
Serine-threonine phosphatase inhibitor 58
Sickle cell disease, test for 162
Simian virus 156
Single stranded deoxyribonucleic acid 55
    fragments 87
Single tissue section 318
Skin 213f
    biopsy 333
    diseases 332
    irritation 132

Slides 228
- adhesives 225, 228
- broken 169
- mounting of 240, 240f, 241
- preparation, monitor quality of 164
- rack 228

Sliding microtome 217, 218
Smooth muscle actin 306, 307f
Smudgy nuclei 262
Sodium
- chloride 189, 300
- citrate buffer 299
- dihydrogen phosphate 188
- dodecyl sulphate polyacrylamide gel electrophoresis 28
- iodate 254, 255
- sulfate 189, 190

Solid-phase extraction 43
- modification of 44
- techniques of 45

Solvent dyes 248
Somatic mutations 11, 15
Southern blotting 76
Specific deoxyribonucleic acid sequence, modification of 34
Specimen 147, 165, 168, 232, 333, 337
- collection of 145
- description 177
- embedding 232
- gross examination of 170
- identification 167
- labeling of 168
- maintain logbook for 169
- orientation of 176
- preparation 316
- rejection, criteria for 169
- retraction facility 220
- shipment of 145
- site 169
- storage of 145
- temperature 233
- test 149
- thickness 206
- types of 145, 154, 177

Spectral color banding technique, development of 32
Spectral karyotyping imaging 31
Spectroscopy 31
Spin column method 43, 44f
Spirit lamp 211
Spraying fixative 183
Squamous epithelium 306
Stainer, integrated system of 260
Staining
- concept of 243
- coupling jars 238
- false negative 327
- false positive 327
- lack of 327
- method 318
- protocol 239, 314, 315f, 338

Standard curve 48, 49f
Staphylococcus
- aureus 137, 156
  - test for 161
- epidermis 137, 156

Sterile
- centrifuge tubes 144
- distilled water 43
- pipette filter tips 143

Stock solution 253, 300
Stomach 306, 307f
Streptococcus
- mutans 156
- pneumoniae, test for 162
- pyogenes 137, 156

Sulfur 245
Surgical procedure, types of 176
Synthesis, next cycle of 90
Synthetic dyes 244

T

T lymphocytes 266
Taq DNA polymerase 77, 90
TaqMan probe 57f, 120
    based assay 55, 61
    based detection 94
    based polymerase chain reaction detection 95f
    based real-time polymerase chain reaction technique 119
    types 56
Target genetic material, helix of 35
Target sequence, flanking regions of 86
Template concentrations 48
Tetramethylrhodamine isothiocynate 279
Thalassemia 24
Thermo fisher 151
Thermus aquaticus 77, 87, 89
Thiazine dyes 245
Thiazole group 245
Three step indirect method 274
Threshold cycle 47, 48f, 93
Tissue 212f, 272-274, 312
    bits 207
    blocks 196
    embedding
        process 207, 211
        system 209
    fixation 165, 177, 282, 329
        technique of 183
    floatation bath 226, 227f
    microarray kits 309f
    orientation of 212, 212f
    over sized chunks of 180f
    over-fixation of 291
    preparation 286
    processing 178, 192, 215
        cassettes for 171f
        cycle, basics of 164f
        schedule 196
    processor 195
    proteins 324
    re-processing of 207
    section 304
    TEK
        base molds 208, 209f
        holder 209f
Toluene 194
Tonsil, normal 326f
Transcending sequencing, perception of 1
Transpathology, concept of 21
Trephine needle 166
Treponema pallidum, test for 162
Triangle shaped tissue lesion 166
Trichloroacetic acid 189
Trichomonas vaginalis 156
    test for 160
Trimming 228
Tris buffer saline 299
Trouble shooting 261, 302, 320
    graphs 62
Tru-cut needle 166
    biopsies 213
Trypsin 292
Tubular structure 213, 213f
Tumor 176f
    cell 15, 306
    identification 231
    solid 4, 86
    types of 163
Tungsten hematoxylin 252
Turn off water bath 298
Two step indirect method 273

Typical thermal cycle might 90
Tyramine amplification 265

U

Ultra-microtome 219
Ultra-rapid dehydration 205
Unique spectral emission, light of 31
Universal nucleic acid extraction kit 126
Unlabeled antibody method 265
Uterus 166
    alveolar rhabdomyosarcoma of 305

V

Vacuum 195, 199, 234
    filtration 45
    function 197
Valid graph 62, 62f
Validates sample integrity 126
Validation chart 312
Van Der Waals force 243, 247
Vapor fixatives 191
Vimentin 306
Viral transmission, risk of 83
Vulva 166

W

Wash biopsy 334
Waste tray 235
Water
    bath 297
        temperature 230
    boiling of 341

Wax
    dispenser 209
    reservoir 209
Wedge biopsy 166
Weigert's iron hematoxylin 253
Western blotting techniques 27, 28, 28f
Whole slide imaging 18
Wooden block 207f

X

Xanthene dyes 245
Xylene 194, 195, 202-204, 215, 243, 261, 287, 338
    changes of 239
    free protocol 205
    miniscule amount of 205

Y

Y-intercept 51, 51f

Z

Zenker's fluid 189, 190
Zenker's formal 190
Zika virus 15
    test for 161, 162
Zinc chloride 188

EU GSPR Authorised Reprsentative
Logos Europe, 9 rue Nicolas Poussin
1700, La Rochelle, France
Phone: +33 (0) 6 67 93 73 78
E-mail: contact@logoseurope.eu

www.ingramcontent.com/pod-product-compliance
Ingram Content Group UK Ltd.
Pitfield, Milton Keynes, MK11 3LW, UK
UKHW022229100725

460641UK00004B/102